LIFESTYLE
MEDICINE Rx

Mr Rush,

I wish you bountiful
blessings, endless joy
and great health.

LIFESTYLE MEDICINE Rx

101 WAYS TO TRANSFORM
YOUR HEALTH AND LIFE

DIANE A. THOMPSON, MD

purposely
created
PUBLISHING

LIFESTYLE MEDICINE RX
Published by Purposely Created Publishing Group™
Copyright © 2019 Diane A. Thompson

All rights reserved.

Printed in the United States of America

ISBN: 978-1-64484-034-4

TABLE OF CONTENTS

INTRODUCTION

Many years ago, as little girl growing up in Jamaica, I believed I would be a teacher and a doctor. I'm uncertain what prompted my interest in teaching—although I have vivid memories of spending endless hours lost in my own world as I pretended to teach the square tiles of the floor in my home—but I'm certain about why I was interested in medicine.

You see, I had asthma as child. My father had it, and I believe at one point I was told my mother did as well. I remember multiple trips to the doctor's office and to Spanish Town Hospital Emergency Room—a small, dark, dingy space with an odd smell and many people looking afraid and desperate—with my then teenage mother. My asthma attacks at their worst would give me the scary feeling of losing each breath, and after each visit to the ER or to my pediatrician's office, I left feeling better—or at least with the knowledge that my mother was given the remedy.

I thought those doctors had some kind of superpower, and I secretly dreamed of one day possessing those powers in order to heal others in the manner that those doctors had healed me.

Although I was a young child, I had some understanding of the class system in Jamaica, and I knew that very few people in my situation could become doctors. I was born to a 16-year-old mother who had brought shame to her family and was thrown out of school and her family home. The prevailing belief at time in Jamaica was that if you made your bed, then you should lie in it. My father was a least 8 years older than my mother, and just two weeks after I made my way into this world, his second child was born to another woman. Pretty soon, he had seven of us born to four different women, and with inconsistent employment and failed businesses, financial support was limited. Jamaican doctors came from a different stock. They were usually from upper-class families with education and connections. I didn't fit that mold, but it didn't stop me from daring to dream.

At age 16, I moved to America, and within weeks of arriving, my mother and I again found ourselves without stable housing. Out of desperation, we both took jobs as live-in housekeepers to ensure we had a place to live, and during our days off, we stayed with friends. In order to get the job, I had to lie to the employer and tell her that I was 20, although I suspect she knew I was only 16. She took advantage of my desperation. I worked for over 70 hours per week cleaning her large home in Westchester County while she paid me less than half the minimum wage. I was promised Saturdays and Sundays off, but I couldn't leave until I again cleaned on Saturday morning, and I had to return by 6 pm on Sundays to prepare her two sons for school. My mom and I both stayed on our respective jobs for a year and saved until we had enough to get our own apartment.

Although a year delayed, I returned to high school at 17, took additional classes in the evenings and during the summer, and excelled. I was able to graduate on time and in the top 1 percent of my class, but since I was initially expected to spend another year to make up for the year I'd missed and no one realized it in time, I missed the prom and the graduation ceremony. There was no celebration or fanfare. My diploma was simply mailed to me.

Based on my grades, I should have had no issues getting into college and then medical school, but I let my 18-year-old mind convince me that it wasn't feasible. I knew I would be the sole provider for my financial needs and for my education, and I was still sorting out my immigration status, so I just couldn't imagine supporting myself through medical school. Since I knew I wanted to help people achieve health and wellness, I thought that if I couldn't go to medical school, then nursing would do.

I graduated from nursing school with honors and received the Theta Sigma Tau Honor Society Award for Clinical Excellence during my graduation from the nurse practitioner program. I then held a series of nursing roles, including staff nurse in the hospital, dermatology nurse in a private office, nurse esthetician, spa nurse, travel nurse, urology nurse practitioner, and adjunct assistant professor of nursing. All that time, though, I yearned to become a doctor. I felt that the additional training and autonomy of being a doctor would allow me to better serve my patients, but as the saying goes, "Good is the enemy of great." It would take more than a decade of nursing before I decided to go after my deferred dream.

While in my 30s, my father passed away from a preventable chronic disease. He was in his 50s and died with most of his own dreams unrealized. I was suddenly aware of my own mortality and decided that life should not be lived with regrets, so I handed in my resignation from my nurse practitioner position, packed my car, and headed from Florida to Pennsylvania.

I excitedly enrolled in a well-known prestigious post-bac premed program and immediately flunked my first general chemistry exam. I was disappointed in myself. After all, I had been an A student. When the instructor asked me to meet with him, I assumed he would comfort me and share the secrets of better study habits. I was dead wrong! Instead, he told me I should immediately drop out of the program and not waste time because I wasn't doctor material and would not get into medical school, and even if I magically managed to get in, I wouldn't survive the first year. He told me I should go back to being a nurse. I wasn't worthy of the attaining the 'superpower'.

I was both sad and embarrassed and cried like a baby. Thankfully, my then-boyfriend, now-husband would have no part of my pity party. He quickly reminded me that someone else's opinion of me is none of my business. He also shared that when someone tells me I can't do something, my only response is to do it and do it well.

I knew this and had even shared this with others whom I had mentored, but in that moment, I needed to be reminded. My husband is smart man, and that's one of the reasons I married him.

I re-learned how to study, and I applied myself. For the rest of that program, I and got As in every class after that first flunk, and after my 8th acceptance to medical school, I stopped interviewing. I was accepted to my first choice of school, graduated, got into my first choice for both internship and residency, was offered a job at the hospital in which I had trained, and within four months of starting the job, I was promoted to Medical Director of the Inpatient Rehabilitation Unit at one of the top hospitals in the country. Indeed, someone's opinion of you is none of your business.

The little poor girl born to a 16-year-old without a solid foundation and expected to fail has grown into an adult who is a triple board-certified medical doctor. I am currently board-certified in physical medicine and rehabilitation, brain injury medicine, and my new passion, lifestyle medicine. I have also attained certifications in health coaching, yoga teacher training, and nutrition. I have done all of these things in order to better position myself to achieve what that little girl with asthma wanted to do so many years ago. I now have the superpower in the form of medical knowledge, personal development techniques, and behavior change strategies, and it allows me to educate and motivate people to make healthy lifestyle changes so they may prevent, halt, and even reverse lifestyle-related diseases.

Over the years, I've watched as many of my own family members die from preventable diseases because they either didn't know lifestyle medicine strategies or knew them but didn't understand how to change their unhealthy behaviors. On a daily basis, I also work with many patients who have found themselves in my rehabilitation unit because of life-style-related diseases. One thing I know for sure about these patients is that no matter how amazing the rehabilitation they've received, it is never as good as not ever having had the disease that brought them there in the first place. This is one of the reasons why what I do is so important.

Dedication

I dedicate my work to my patients as well as my many family members who have died prematurely of lifestyle-related ill-nesses. This includes my father and my maternal grandfather, who both died in their 50s from preventable cardiopulmo-nary disease; my sweet uncle and my grandmother, who both suffered with high blood pressure and diabetes along with the many sequelae of diabetes; and my once active grandaunt who now lives with dementia as well as a leg amputation and blindness courtesy of diabetes. I will work to spread the word because I realize that health is truly wealth, and I am in a unique position to help people maintain their health.

This book shares information and strategies used by people all over the world to help you take control of your health and to help you live a longer and happier life. Some of these practices have been backed by strong scientific evidence, while others are shared mainly from tradition or anecdotes. Some are commonly practiced in the United States, while others are better known in foreign lands.

I wish you great health.

Why Lifestyle Medicine?

Lifestyle medicine is one of the most exciting and emerging fields in medicine that equips you with the knowledge, tools, and power to control your health, boost wellness, and enhance happiness through evidence-based lifestyle interventions. Lifestyle medicine offers help to reduce the risk of diseases, manage health conditions, and even reverse some diseases.

Over the years, medicine has focused on conventional methods of managing and treating chronic diseases by mostly offering a temporary fix after the disease is already present, with a goal of controlling the symptoms. You have high blood pressure or diabetes? You'd get an anti-hypertensive or diabetes pill, and it is generally expected that with time you would need more or other medications to treat these chronic diseases. In addition, since you haven't necessarily addressed the disease itself, you are at risk of getting other diseases that result from the underlying disease. It seems it is a no-win situation for you as the consumer of healthcare. If you remain with the chronic disease for the rest of your life, our current health care system and the pharmaceutical giants continue to win. You, on the other hand, may not get to live your life with the quality it deserves. Keeping you a patient for the rest of your life was not why I decided to become a doctor. I became a doctor to help you TRANSFORM your health. (More on this acronym shortly.)

In my own family, just about everyone has diabetes. A few years ago, when I wasn't paying attention to my own health and developed pre-diabetes, I used lifestyle medicine strategies to reverse it. In this book, I presented 101 simple practices that have been shown to help prevent chronic health problems, manage current diseases, and even reverse some of them. There are also wellness practices to help with your fitness, happiness, stress level, and self-care.

Get ready to TRANSFORM!

Disclaimer

The goal is to educate you about lifestyle medicine principles and wellness practices and allow you to discuss them with your doctor so that the both of you in partnership may decide which practices may be helpful or beneficial for you. This book is not intended to be used for diagnosis or treatment and does not establish a doctor-patient relationship with the author.

TRANSFORM

CHAPTER 1

Take Stock and
Take Back

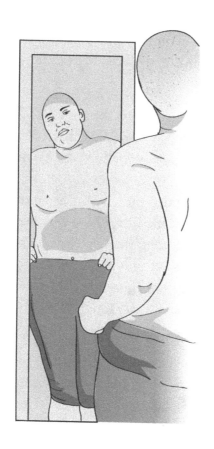

*You can't really know where you are going
until you know where you've been.*

~**Maya Angelou**

I. MANAGE YOUR MINDSET AND MAKE A MINDSET SHIFT

You, like billions of people worldwide, have probably participated in the New Year's ritual of resolution setting. And before the month of January is over, you, and the majority of those people, have consistently failed to execute.

One of the biggest reasons for this is that change in behavior is generally preceded by a mindset shift. Many people who pack the gyms on New Year's Day have done so many times before and have consistently not stuck with their plan because they entered the New Year with the same mindset as the year before and ended up with the same results. Americans are also the unhealthiest they have ever been despite having easy access to health information. This suggests that a lack of healthy behavior is not simply due to a lack of information. In fact, many people who engage in risky or unhealthy lifestyle behaviors are generally very much aware of the risks.

So, what do you need to do to ensure this time will be different? You need to assess your mindset and make a mindset shift. If you've had trouble with overeating or eating unhealthy foods, assess what beliefs you have around food. Do you eat food for comfort or do see food as a vehicle to provide nutrients to enable you to live your best life? Your view will determine what you choose to eat.

What are your beliefs around being overweight? One client told me that since everyone in her family was overweight she viewed herself as normal, and during the times she considered losing weight because she could barely walk one flight of stairs and was now diabetic, she wondered if her family would view her differently. She didn't want to be different, even if it meant an early death. Your view of being overweight, like that of my client, will determine whether or not you chose to do anything about it.

Do you feel you are deserving of great health? If you don't believe you are deserving, you are not likely to do the work it takes to achieve it.

Another step is to look at past failures. Are you some-one who has lost and regained weight many times before? It's possible that after a few times you have adopted the mindset that you are going to fail, and this then becomes a self-full-ing prophesy. Before embarking on this or any life-changing journey, get out your journal and determine what you want to change, then do an assessment of your mindset around that subject. It may be time to manage your mindset and make a mindset shift.

2.   ASSESS YOUR READINESS FOR CHANGE

After speaking at dozens of events and coaching and consulting with thousands of people, I can accurately say no one will change until they are ready. Scientists have studied behavior change for centuries, and various behavior change models tend to support this. The Transtheoretical Model of Behavior Change looks at the stages of behavior change, and where someone is on that continuum can accurately predict whether or not that person will have success with changing his or her behavior. The stage a person is in will also determine the best strategies to help them move along and reach success in achieving their goals.

Stages of Change:

▶ Precontemplation: The person does not intend to make changes anytime soon.

▶ Contemplation: The person intends to make the change in about the next six months.

▶ Preparation (Determination): The person is ready to take action within the next 30 days.

▶ Action: The person has changed behavior and intends to move forward.

▶ Maintenance: The person has sustained the behavior change and intends to maintain it.

▶ Termination: The person has no desire to return to the unhealthy behavior.

As you can see, success in your health will be different based on the stage you are in when you are attempting to make the change. The resources offered to a smoker who is not ready to stop smoking are very different from those offered to someone who has stopped but occasionally smokes during times of stress. So before attempting the change, determine where you are in the process, since the support you need to help you succeed will be different.

3. TAKE AN ASSESSMENT OF YOUR HEALTH

A few years ago, I went to my primary care doctor for a routine physical only to find out that I was not only 15 pounds heavier than I had been the year before, but also that my hemoglobin A1C—a measure of your blood sugar over several weeks—was now 6.4 (up from 4.9 the year before), placing me in the pre-diabetic category.

Since I had been skinny all my life—in fact, I am now embarrassed to admit that during my teenage years I commonly took weight gain supplements—and had never had a chronic disease, I didn't take the new diagnosis seriously.

I continued with my usual clinical practice of seeing patients, my administrative role of medical director, my academic work of educating medical students and residents, and my volunteer work of providing health education for the community, and I didn't take heed to the saying, "Physician, heal thyself." Three months later, a re-assessment revealed I was exactly where I had been three months earlier. Nothing changed until I decided to take stock of what I was doing wrong and took the necessary steps to take back my health.

One of the best strategies for achieving success in your health goals is to take an assessment of where you are, what got you there, and what tools you need to in order to improve your health. Once I did that, I realized I had developed the habit of working late nights in my office in order to complete my notes. On those late evenings I would comfort and reward myself with a cup of tea, and of course, you can't have tea without a pastry. Pretty soon, I had developed this additional 400-calorie-a-day habit, and since I was working late, it meant I would have no time for exercise. Once I knew the problem, I knew exactly what needed to change, and six months later, I lost most of the weight and reversed the pre-diabetes.

10 Questions to Ask Before Starting Your Health Journey:

▶ What are your goals?

▶ Why do you want these goals? You must know your why.

▶ What will change if you achieve this goal?

▶ What are some reasons you haven't yet achieved this goal?

▶ What started your journey into an unhealthy lifestyle?

▶ When were the times you were successful in achieving goals in the past?

▶ What strategies did you employ to achieve success during those times?

▶ Who will be a part of your support system?

▶ When were the times you failed at executing a plan?

▶ What contributed to those failures and what strategies did you use to recover?

4.   EAT TO LIVE INSTEAD OF LIVING TO EAT

People sometimes think that practicing healthy living is difficult, but one of the strategic steps in order to be successful with major change is to change your mindset around why we eat. Indeed, unhealthy foods can sometimes look and smell better and are even designed to be more delicious. Once you understand that food represents fuel and consuming quality food will enable you to perform at your best, it becomes less challenging to select food that supports your health.

That said, there are ways to make healthy food taste good and present well, and this may require another mindset shift around how you prepare and serve the food. Another mindset shift may need to occur around the fact that healthy living is a lifestyle and not just a temporary fix. Once you accept that you need to eat to live, you begin to find strategies to sustain your new healthy lifestyle.

5.   KNOW YOUR NUMBERS

Some of the most important numbers you need to know in order to take control of your health are your blood pressure, cholesterol, high density lipoprotein (HDL) (or healthy cholesterol), low density lipoprotein (LDL) (or lousy lipids), weight, abdominal circumference, body mass index (BMI), and hemoglobin A1C. Based on your specific medical condition, there are other numbers that may also be important to your health, so check with your doctor. Once you know these numbers, you can determine what lifestyle changes you need to make.

6.   LEARN WAYS TO CONTROL YOUR BLOOD PRESSURE

First know the number, then understand the risks associated with high blood pressure (also known as hypertension). High blood pressure puts you at risk for many diseases, including stroke, and is considered a modifiable risk factor, meaning you can change it.

Some strategies for reducing high blood pressure include reducing your sodium or salt intake, eating a whole food plant-based diet, eating potassium-rich foods, consuming foods known to improve high blood pressure, reducing your stress, reducing your weight, and exercising.

5 Foods Shown to Help Reduce Blood Pressure:

▶ Whole food plant-based (WFPB) diet

▶ Hibiscus (often consumed as a drink or tea)

▶ Beets

▶ Pomegranates

▶ Flaxseeds

According to WebMD, potassium-rich foods include:

▶ Bananas

▶ Oranges

▶ Cantaloupe

▶ Honeydew

▶ Apricots

▶ Grapefruit

▶ Dried fruits (such as prunes, raisins, and dates)

▶ Cooked spinach

▶ Cooked broccoli

▶ Potatoes

▶ Sweet potatoes

▶ Mushrooms

▶ Peas

▶ Cucumbers

7. UNDERSTAND YOUR OPTIMAL WEIGHT

Various diseases have been associated with being overweight and obese. It is often said that it is not how much a person weighs that is important to their health, it's how much fat they have. BMI, or body mass index, is an approximation of a person's fatness. This is calculated by taking the person's weight in kilograms divided by the square of the height in meters. There are also free BMI calculators available online, including at the National Institute of Health (NIH) https://www.nhlbi.nih.gov/health/educational/lose_wt/BMI/bmicalc.htm

Determining where you lie in the BMI categories will help to know if you need to gain, maintain, or lose weight. Although there are people who are underweight, the vast majority of Americans fall in the overweight or obese categories.

BMI Categories

Underweight = <18.5

Normal Weight = 18.5-24.9

Overweight = 25-29.9

Obesity = BMI of 30 or greater

10 Strategies to Help with Weight Loss:

▶ Center your meals around plants (whole food plant-based).

▶ Choose foods that are high in nutrients and lower in calories.

▶ Eat foods that keep you feeling full, such as beans or oats.

▶ Avoid high-calorie processed foods, such as white breads, pastries, or cookies.

▶ Avoid liquid calories in the form of sodas and juices.

▶ Avoid late-night eating.

▶ Have healthier food options, such as fruits and vegetables, readily available.

▶ Avoid unhealthy snacking.

▶ Pay attention to your portion sizes. Are you eating enough for two people?

▶ Add exericse to your daily routine.

8.   PRACTICE GOOD TIME MANAGEMENT

Poor time management can reflect itself in increased stress and may limit your ability to maintain good lifestyle medicine and wellness practices. It is well known that the number-one reason people give for not exercising or eating healthful is lack of time. You can make a major difference in your perception of the time you have just by implementing simple time management strategies.

10 Simple but Effective Time Management Tips:

▶ Plan your day the night before.

▶ Get up one hour earlier.

▶ Have a morning routine (read *Miracle Mornings* for suggestions).

▶ Focus on one goal at a time.

▶ Avoid multitasking.

▶ Take a social media fast.

▶ Batch tasks so that similar tasks are done at the same time.

▸ Get a good night sleep so that you are performing at your best.

▸ Get comfortable at delegating.

▸ Use an organizing app or a planner.

9. WILLPOWER ALONE IS NOT ENOUGH

One of the simplest steps to ensure you eat healthily is to ensure that healthy foods are readily available in your home or work space. If you plan to use willpower as your main strategy to attain and maintain health, you are setting up yourself for failure.

Your body aims to keep your weight at a certain set point, so sometimes when you have lost weight, you may notice that there is an urge to eat more to get back to the original weight. I experienced this when I lost the 15 pounds that contributed to me being pre-diabetic. There are also reward systems in the brain, and it is safe to say most people will be more tempted by a slice of cake than a cup of broccoli. Some studies have suggested that if you have spent much of the morning resisting many temptations, by the end of the day, your willpower has a will of its own, and you are likely to give in. Sadness and loneliness may also make it difficult to resist certain temptations.

To increase your chance of success, ensure that your refrigerator and pantry are stocked with healthy food options and pack healthy foods to take with you to work. Replace unhealthy snacks and ensure that your environment and work space match your goal of attaining a healthier lifestyle. Don't just rely on willpower to achieve success because willpower will fail you.

10. THE SECRET WEAPON OF THE ACCOUNTABILITY BUDDY

I recently started business coaching, and one of the best parts of the program is that each person is paired up with another person so that we can keep each other accountable. The organizer probably knew of the findings that suggest that this type of support from someone who is similarly in the trenches can help you get further faster. You can't fly like an eagle if you hang out with pigeons. This partner or accountability buddy can be used in a similar way to help keep you honest in your health journey. Your accountability partner can check in to ensure you are on track and may offer encouragement for those moments that you need them.

10 Other Benefits of an Accountability Partner:

▶ They can be your cheerleader.

▶ They can be a source of motivation.

▶ They can help you manage your feeling of overwhelm.

▶ They can help you keep the main thing the main thing.

▶ They can offer a different perspective.

▸ They can provide emotional support.

▸ They can be sources of information.

▸ They can provide challenges.

▸ They can encourage your growth.

▸ They can keep you in momentum.

II. TAKE FULL RESPONSIBILITY

I was the product of a teenage pregnancy. My mom was pregnant with me at the age of 15, and back then, many Jamaican parents dealt with this embarrassment by putting the offender—in this case the teen mother—out to fend for herself. The common saying was "If you make the bed, lie in it," so this act was seen as teaching the teen mother a lesson. No one gave much thought to the fact that a fifteen-year-old unemployed high school dropout was not equipped to take care of a child and that adding being homeless to that mix was not teaching anyone a lesson but simply ensuring failure for all involved.

Such a difficult start in my life resulted in many challenges in the earlier part of my life, but despite those struggles, I was able to accomplish many of my dreams. One of the main reasons for this is that I took full responsibility for where I was and for what I wanted to achieve.

The moment you decide to take full responsibility for where you are in your health, despite early poor nutrition, low nutritional education, or even the genes you've inherited, is the moment you have the potential to take control of your health and make the necessary changes. If you continue to blame others for where you are, you won't give yourself the chance to live up to your highest potential. Your brain is waiting for you to tell it to find the solutions. This rings true when it comes to health, finances, relationships, career, or anything important to you. Take full responsibility for where you are. That's the only way you will find your solution to a way out.

12. LEARN FROM THE PEOPLE IN THE BLUE ZONES

There is a saying that goes, "success leaves clues," and the lifestyle of the people of the Blue Zones—the five regions in the world with the highest concentration of people who live much healthier and longer lives than average—gives an abundance of evidence about the life-transforming effects of implementing lifestyle medicine strategies in our lives.

The five regions are Okinawa, Japan; Sardinia, Italy; Nicoya, Costa Rica; Icaria, Greece; and Loma Linda, California (particularly among the Seventh-Day Adventist population there).

Study of these populations revealed that people in the Blue Zones share common lifestyle practices that are believed to contribute to their health and longevity.

8 Blue Zone Practices:

▶ Plant-Based Nutrition: The majority of food consumed by these people comes from plants.

▶ A Love of Legumes: Beans make up a significant portion of their foods.

▶ Family Focus: Family and relationships are integral to their way of life.

▶ Connectedness: Social interaction and a sense of community are paramount.

▶ Smoking avoidance

▶ Physical Activity: They don't necessarily join gyms but find ways to remain physically active.

▶ Moderate alcohol intake

▶ A sense of purpose

13. DECLUTTER YOUR ENVIRONMENT

It has been reported that cleaning up creates a sense of confidence and self-efficacy, improves creativity, reduces anxiety, increases your energy, limits time wasting, and helps reduce financial stress. These benefits may also help you on your health journey and contribute to your wellness.

10 Successful De-Cluttering Tips:

▶ Figure out your style: Do you accomplish things fast and furious or slow and steady?

▶ The power of focus: Attacking one drawer or one area first may improve your confidence.

▶ Schedule a specific time for cleanup.

▶ Determine if you are holding on to something for emotional or sentimental reasons.

▶ If you haven't worn a piece of clothing in a year, someone else can benefit from it.

▶ Ask for help so you don't feel overwhelmed.

▶ Everything should have a home.

▶ Don't beat up on yourself if you haven't seen much progress.

▶ Take before and after photos to track your progress and to feel accomplished.

▶ Reward yourself after each area has been cleaned.

14. TAKE ADVANTAGE OF YOUR EMPLOYEE WELLNESS PROGRAM

Are you having trouble staying healthy on your own? As mentioned above, support can make all the difference. This support may come from the most unexpected place, such as your employee wellness program or even a health ministry in your church.

Many companies now offer wellness checks, challenges, and group health programs. Others allow employees to use pre-tax money towards health coaching or health groups. Check with your human resources department, and if there isn't a wellness program, perhaps you can start one. There are many like-minded people in your organization who are also looking for help and support to improve their health.

THINGS TO HELP ME TRANSFORM

THINGS TO HELP ME TRANSFORM

THINGS TO HELP ME TRANSFORM

THINGS TO HELP ME TRANSFORM

_____

_____

_____

_____

_____

_____

_____

_____

_____

_____

_____

_____

_____

_____

_____

CHAPTER 2

Rest and Relaxation

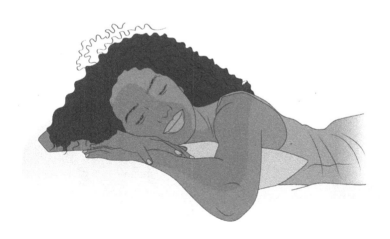

Sometimes the most urgent thing you can
possibly do is to take a complete rest.
~**Ashleigh Brilliant**

15. BREATHE

It is believed that deep breathing has the potential to help relieve tension, improve circulation, and even reduce insomnia. Many practitioners of yoga believe that this deep breathing as practiced by yogis produces a sensation of heat, calms the body, strengthens the respiratory system, soothes the nervous system, and reduces craving. Breathing can take the form of simply breathing in through the nose for a count of 10 and out through the mouth for the same count, or it can me more involved, such as the 4-7-8 technique as taught by Dr. Andrew Weil, a physician and integrative medicine practitioner.

According to Dr. Weil's website, in this particular breathing technique, the practitioner places the tip of the tongue against the skin just behind the top of the front teeth, then begins by exhaling completely through the mouth making a "whoosh" sound. The mouth is then closed and the breath is inhaled quietly through the nose to a count of four. The breath is held for a count of seven, then exhaled completely though the mouth making the same "whoosh" sound for a count of eight. This is often repeated two to three times. Practitioners are advised that with initial practice, lightheadedness may be experienced, but it tends to improve as they get acclimated to this type of breathing.

Whatever technique you choose, know that with breathing, you have a simple yet powerful tool that may be used anywhere and at any time to help reset your mood, provide relaxation, or decrease stress.

16. ACUPUNCTURE

Acupuncture has been practiced in China for at least 2,500 years. Although there are now variations to the practice, it generally involves inserting very thin needles into the skin in specific areas of the body. Traditional Chinese medicine describes acupuncture as a way to balance the flow of energy in your body. In Western medicine, acupuncture is often used in pain management.

There are many claims made by some practitioners of acupuncture that have not yet been shown by research, so if you choose to include this in your wellness practices, do your research and speak with your physician. Acupuncture should only be done by a trained specialist, and treatments may be covered by your insurance.

10 Reasons People Use Acupuncture:

▶ Headache relief

▶ Stress relief

▸ Immune function improvement

▸ Allergy relief

▸ Relief from digestive conditions

▸ Eye strain relief

▸ Improved energy

▸ Cigarette craving reduction

▸ Weight loss

▸ Anti-aging

17. BUY A GOOD MATTRESS

A good mattress can help prevent several pain issues, such as lower back and neck pain. According to the National Sleep Foundation, a mattress has a lifespan of approximately eight years. Depending on the quality and type of your mattress, you may get more or less time from it. Any mattress made with higher quality material is likely going to last longer, and the type of mattress you buy makes a difference.

Innerspring: An innerspring mattress contains a coil support system that helps to distribute your weight evenly across mattress. They can last up to 10 years or sometimes longer if they are two-sided and can be flipped over for more evenly distributed wear and tear.

Memory Foam: A memory foam mattress comes in different materials and densities, which will determine how well it holds up. A quality memory foam mattress can last from 10 to 15 years with the right care.

18. SLEEP HYGIENE

The current finding is that most Americans don't get an adequate amount of sleep, which leads to daytime sleepiness, mood and performance impairment, poor reaction time and driving performance, and memory deficits. In fact, a lack of sleep may result in numerous emotional and physical issues, and a sleep-deprived person performs in a similar way an intoxicated person does. Sleep deprivation can have a negative impact on all organ systems in the body. Another interesting finding is that you are unable to make up on the weekends for poor sleep during the week.

Good sleep habits (sometimes referred to as "sleep hygiene") can help you get a good night's sleep. To ensure good health, you must get adequate and deep restful and restorative sleep. Although no official guideline for sleep exists, several organizations suggest that adults need seven to nine hours and teens about nine to ten hours of sleep per night.

10 Strategies for Improved Sleep:

▶ Set a bedtime and wakeup time the same time every day.

▶ Avoid caffeinated beverages.

▸ Avoid alcohol before sleep.

▸ Avoid large meals before bed.

▸ Remove electronic devices such as smart phones, TVs, and computers from the bedroom.

▸ Designate the bedroom as a place for sex and sleep.

▸ Exercise, but avoid doing so close to bedtime.

▸ Keep the bedroom quiet, dark, and cool.

▸ Have a ritual before bedtime to train your brain for sleep.

▸ Get clearance from your physician before deciding to take a sleep aid.

19. ASSESS FOR TENSION

Are you tense? Try to relax your body to see if there are signs of tension. Is your body relaxed or rigid? Can your jaws open up freely? Do your hands fall freely to your sides? Take note to see where there is tension in your body and take steps to relive it.

10 Strategies for Dealing with Tension:

▸ Get a massage.

▸ Practice actively relaxing every part of the body from toe to head.

▸ Take a warm bath.

▸ Do some gentle stretching.

▸ Get adequate and deep restorative sleep.

▸ Practice deep breathing techniques.

▸ Go for a walk.

▸ Practice meditation.

▸ Eat healthily by increasing plant-based foods.

▸ Keep yourself hydrated.

20. SCHEDULE TIME TO DECOMPRESS

Setting aside a few minutes for yourself can help rejuvenate your mind and body. Find moments to be alone. This may mean locking yourself away in the bathroom for five minutes where you can practice deep breathing and meditation or take longer and indulge in a warm bath.

10 Strategies to Find Time to Decompress:

▸ Make an assessment of how you spend your time.

▸ Schedule time with yourself.

▸ Delegate.

▸ Remember that "No" is a complete sentence.

▶ Declutter your schedule.

▶ Use your commute time for relaxing.

▶ Take a break from electronics.

▶ Take a break from social media.

▶ Take a nap.

▶ Enjoy your shower.

21. MASSAGE THERAPY

Massage is a term used to describe manipulating the skin, muscles, ligament, and tendons, and includes a variety of interactions such as light stoking, tapping, or deep pressure. Initially, massage was seen more as a part of integrative or complementary medicine. Today, the benefits are better appreciated, and the practice is now commonly seen in doctor's offices, health clinics, spas, gyms, and even airports.

Although practitioners of massage therapy generally report the benefits, it is important to recognize that some patients may be at increased risks of injury. Therefore, you should consider getting clearance from your physician prior to participating in massage. Patients at increased risk of injury during massage include those on blood thinners and those who have thrombocytopenia or low platelets, an active infection, open wounds, deep vein thrombosis (clot), and severe osteoporosis.

4 Massage Types:

▸ Trigger Point Massage: This type of massage focuses on loosening tight, sometimes painful, muscle bands and trigger points.

▸ Swedish Massage: This is a gentle massage that involves stroking, tapping, and rubbing with a goal of stress and tension reduction and relaxation.

▸ Deep Tissues Massage: This is a more intense massage that aims to get to the deeper tissue to address injuries.

▸ Sports Massage: This is aimed at athletes or sports performers to help prevent injuries.

10 Reported Benefits of Massage:

▸ Promotes relaxation

▸ Reduces stress

▸ Relives anxiety

▸ Improves generalized body aches and pain

▸ Relieves headaches

▸ Improves sleep

▶ Relive sports injuries

▶ Addresses temporomandibular joint (TMJ)-related pain

▶ Helps with discomfort from fibromyalgia

▶ Relieves digestive disorders

5 Reported Risks Associated with Massage Therapy:

▶ Bruising

▶ Discomfort, especially with deep tissue massage

▶ Bleeding, especially if you are on blood thinners

▶ Fractures, especially in people with osteoporosis

▶ Deep vein thrombosis or clot

5 Questions to Ask Your Massage Therapist:

▶ Are you licensed to perform massages?

▶ What is your training?

▶ For how long have you been performing massages?

▶ Is your massage covered by insurance?

▶ How many sessions will you need?

7 Ways to Locate a Massage Therapist:

▸ Ask your physician or a friend for recommendations

▸ Look for referrals at local massage therapy schools

▸ Look for therapists at the American Massage Therapy Association (AMTA) website

▸ Browse the Alliance of Massage Therapy Education website: https://www.afmte.org/

▸ Browse the Massage Therapy Foundation website: http://massagetherapyfoundation.org/

▸ Look for a provider on the Board Certification in Therapeutic Massage and Body Work (BCTMB) website: https://www.ncbtmb.org/

▸ Browse the Associated Bodywork and Massage Professional website: https://www.abmp.com/

22. SELF-MASSAGE

Self-massage is, as the name states, the practice of massaging your own body parts with your own hands or with tools. People who practice self-massage see it as a convenient and inexpensive way to relieve pain, tension, and stress.

8 Tools Commonly Used During Self-Massage:

▶ Foam roller

▶ Trigger point cane

▶ Back buddy

▶ Rolling stick

▶ Tennis ball

▶ Theraband foot roller

▶ Motor massage cushion

▶ Massage chair

23. BODY SCRUB

A body scrub is often seen as a way of mechanically exfoliating the skin with the goal of stimulating circulation and removing dead cells in order to reveal newer, more youthful looking skin. Scrubs may be purchased or can be made using a variety of recipes.

5 Reported Benefits of Body Scrubs:

▶ Appearance of smoother skin

▶ Reduced appearance of acne

▶ Reduced appearance of dark spots

▶ Helps prevents ingrown hairs

▶ Stress reduction

Honey and Oatmeal Body Scrub Recipe:

▶ ½ cup oatmeal

▶ 2 tablespoons honey

▶ 2 tablespoons course cornmeal

▶ 2 tablespoons apple cider vinegar

▶ 2 tablespoons coconut oil

▶ Apply all ingredients in glass bowls and mix until you get a paste-like consistency.

▶ Apply paste in bathroom and rub briskly. Rinse off with warm water followed by moisturizer.

24. GONG

Gong therapy, also known as gong sound therapy or gong bath, is seen as a sound massage for the mind and body. This therapy uses metal percussion instruments (gongs), which produce sounds during therapy, prayer, ritual, and meditation. Practitioners describe the benefits of this sounds therapy as being conducive to relaxation, producing a sense of centering, and facilitating the healing process.

In general, classes may begin with the instructor setting a mantra to help the participant center and quiet their minds. Sessions may be mixed with elements of yoga as well as reiki and typically last thirty minutes to an hour and a half. Gongs are then played by the instructor and use vibrational frequency, which helps some people go into a deep state of sleep and relaxation.

As of this writing, there are no clinical trials showing that this particular sound therapy works, but some practitioners liken it to music therapy. Studies suggest that music therapy can help to decrease stress, improve relaxation, and lower blood pressure.

25. LIGHT THERAPY

Light therapy, also used to treat some skin disorders, has been commonly used to help disorders such as Seasonal Affective Disorder (SAD), a type of depression that is generally seen during the winter months.

Since there are possible adverse effects associated with the use of light therapy, consult with your doctor before trying this therapy.

5 Conditions Treated with Light Therapy:

▶ Seasonal Affective Disorder (SAD)

▶ Sleep disorders

- Jetlag

- Dementia

- Circadian rhythm disorders in shift workers

26. ART THERAPY

Art therapy includes activities such as sculpting, drawing, painting, woodworking, ceramics, quilting, and pottery. Research studies support the idea that creating art may help facilitate great health and may have similar health benefits to regular exercise, meditation, and a balanced nutrition. A review of the literature shows specific benefits such as stress reduction, reduction of depressive symptoms, improved immune functioning, and enhanced positive emotions. Patients who may find benefits from art therapy include those with dementia, cancer, and Parkinson's disease. It is even believed that the viewer of the art may experience a similar impact as the creator.

27. THE BENEFITS OF BATHS

Bathing is not just for personal hygiene but has been also found to have stress-reducing and wellness benefits for the mind and body.

Hot baths could result in burns as well as heart issues in persons with pre-existing heart disease.

5 Reported Benefits of Baths:

▶ Improved breathing and reduced decongestion, especially if you add eucalyptus

▶ Reduced pain and inflammation of the muscles

▶ Improved circulation

▶ Relaxation

▶ Improved sleep

28. JUST RELAX

The demands of life can make stress inevitable, but it doesn't have to be so. Learn to be present. Practice relaxation techniques to help focus and center your mind. Life can be hectic, but you don't need to be. So clear your schedule and just relax.

5 Strategies for Relaxation:

▶ Take slow, deep breaths

▶ Take a warm bath

▶ Practice guided imagery

▶ Meditate

▶ Practice self-massage

29.   MANAGE YOUR STRESS

Stress occurs when our perception of our problems seems bigger than our coping abilities. Stress is not necessarily a negative thing, but chronic stress, especially when the individual feels out of control, can be very damaging to the health and is known to negatively affect just about every system in the body. Take the necessary steps to acknowledge and manage your stress.

10 Strategies for Stress Reduction:

▶   Identify your stressor

▶   Change the way you view stress

▶   Avoid stressful situations

▶   Journal

▶   Exercise regularly

▶   Eat a whole food plant-based diet

▶   Meditate

▶   Get social support

▶   Smile

▶   Get adequate sleep

30. LEARN TO DELEGATE

For people who take pride in their responsibilities and who are passionate about what they do, the act of delegating can be seen as a no-no. But entrusting others with responsibilities that would normally fill your time and energy may be one of the quickest ways to self-actualization. Not only does delegating have the potential to empower someone else, but it also allows you to better manage your time, increase your efficiency, and cultivate your creativity. It also allows you the freedom to focus on the things you are best at and the things that matters most.

31. NO PROBLEM, MON!

When I was a child growing up in Jamaica, a common saying among the natives was "No problem, mon!" It didn't matter if that person had very little, they would make do with what they had and live with the view that tomorrow offered another day and more opportunities.

Today, when people are chronically exposed to the damaging effects of stress, this may be a good attitude to adopt. Take stock of what is causing you stress and immediately change the things you can. For the things out of your control, remember "No problem, mon," and don't sweat the small stuff.

32. RECOGNIZE BURNOUT AND ADDRESS IT

Do you please others at the detriment of yourself? Are you experiencing the effects of burnout?

A couple of years after starting my job as a physician, I realized that I went to work early in the mornings, stayed late in the evenings to finish notes, didn't get enough sleep, ate poorly, and spent much of my weekends cleaning and running errands only to return to work on Mondays as tired as I was on Fridays. I realized that I was suffering from the beginning stages of burnout, and my solution was to cut back on my time at work.

If you are suffering from burnout, stop and assess ways in which you are able to better address your work, schedule, and family life. Take steps to take care of your mind and body, eat nutritious food, enjoy good times with loved ones, and have a life outside of work.

5 Signs of Burnout

▶ Insomnia: In the early stages of burnout, you may notice that you have trouble falling asleep or staying asleep. As burnout persists, you might have chronic insomnia even while you are tired. Many people put a Band-Aid on the problem by taking a sleep aid, and since the reason for the burnout has not been addressed, any attempts at implementing good sleep hygiene may prove ineffective.

▶ Fatigue: Some people may experience fatigue early on, but as burnout is allowed to progress without appropriate intervention, they may find themselves feeling exhausted and unable to function.

▶ Appetite Changes: It is not uncommon for people who are experiencing burnout to eat less or eat more. Those eating less may end up not receiving the proper nutrients, and those overeating may often find that they reach for "comfort food" which are oftentimes laden with sugar, salt, and unhealthy fats and are low in nutrients. Either way, this is a recipe for poor health and wellness.

▶ Inattention and Poor Concentration: Burnout may lead people to have decreased concentration, which may show itself as decreased attention to details and poor memory. These cognitive impairments may also be magnified in persons who are also not eating or sleeping well. If allowed to progress, quality of work and relationships may be negatively impacted, which can contribute to mood changes.

▶ Mood Changes: As burnout is allowed to progress without intervention, the person may feel out of control, and this may lead to anxiety and depression, which could further impact work and relationships and worsen the situation.

10 Strategies to Handle Burnout and Protect Your Health:

▶ Nourish your body with healthy foods. Aim for at least five to seven servings of fruits and vegetables.

▶ Hydrate yourself. Unless you have been restricted by your doctor, hydrate yourself with plain water and avoid sugary beverages.

▶ Get enough sleep.

▶ Exercise regularly.

▶ Recognize early burnout signs and don't ignore them. Begin to address them early on.

▶ Just say no. If you try to become everything to everyone, you risk becoming nothing to everyone. More importantly, you increase your likelihood of becoming ill.

▶ Figure out strategies and outlets that tend to work for you and have them ready. Some people find that solitude, prayer, or meditation helps, while others want a crowd around them during times of stress. Find what works for you and work it.

▶ Assess how you are when things are good and when things are not. This allows you to recognize early signs of burnout so you have the best chance of beating it.

▶ Put down your superhero cape and ask for help. Acknowledging that you need help is actually a sign of strength and maturity and not a sign of weakness.

▶ Surround yourself with positive people. Many times, the perspective of the people around us can determine how we process a situation. Find yourself a couple of positive Pamelas or Percys and have them on speed dial.

▶ Don't be afraid to seek professional help.

33. PRACTICE THE COUNTDOWN TECHNIQUE

This involves counting down from ten to zero. Take a complete deep breath with each number you count all the way to zero. You can repeat as slowly or as fast as you like. This practice can be done anytime and as many times as you like. This allows you to reset and calm yourself.

THINGS TO HELP ME TRANSFORM

THINGS TO HELP ME TRANSFORM

THINGS TO HELP ME TRANSFORM

THINGS TO HELP ME TRANSFORM

_____

_____

_____

_____

_____

_____

_____

_____

_____

_____

_____

_____

_____

_____

_____

_____

CHAPTER 3

Appreciate

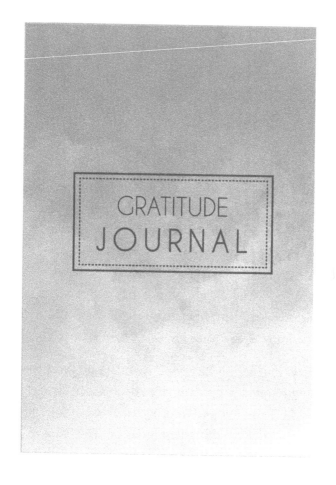

A grateful heart is a magnet for miracles.
~**Unknown**

34. CULTIVATE AN ATTITUDE OF GRATITUDE

People who are grateful tend to be happier and less stressed, but they were not necessarily blessed with this attribute. Instead, most people who are grateful tend to cultivate the attitude. In fact, why should the universe bless you with things you want when you haven't learned to appreciate the things you already have? So begin cultivating an attitude of gratitude by actively looking for things for which you should be thankful.

35. GRATITUDE JOURNAL

I started journaling many years ago as a teenager, back when it was called "writing in a diary." Back then, I was a loner and shy, and my mother and I didn't have the best relationship. My journal offered me an outlet where I felt free to share my thoughts and an avenue to release my pent-up feelings. In fact, I am so passionate about journaling that many years ago I created the "Healthy Inspirations" journals and included a gratitude journal in the series.

Today, journaling has gone mainstream, and there have been documented benefits such as decrease in stress level, depression, and anxiety, and improvement in happiness level. As the saying goes, "Anything you focus on, you expand." So it is not hard to believe that when journaling is used to focus on gratitude, the person journaling tends to feel more grateful.

10 Reported Benefits of Journaling:

▸ Enhances wellbeing

▸ Manages anxiety

▸ Reduces stress

▸ Helps with goal setting

▸ Tracks your progress

▸ Helps with focus

▸ Improves cognitive functioning

▸ Strengthens the immune system

▸ Improves creativity

▸ Helps to cultivate gratitude

36.   SHORE UP YOUR SUPPORT SYSTEM

Life comes with hills and valleys. Having a community of like-minded people during the down times may help manage the low moments and even decrease the amount of time spent there. A support system can also provide a sense of connection and lets you know you are not alone. Often, someone in your support system may offer you a different perspective on handling your stress. The key to having an effective support system is to not wait until you are in need of them to identify them.

5 Tips to Get Support:

▶ Identify and create your support network and build a relationship before you need them.

▶ Offer yourself as support to someone else.

▶ Recognize that support systems can be found in typical locations such as your place of worship, but also in atypical places like online groups or within social groups. For example, my social support includes friends I met in Toastmasters from years earlier, colleagues in my coaching group, and even people I met on social media.

▶ Limit your interactions with negative people.

▶ Don't be afraid to ask for help when you need it.

37. MAKE YOUR MORNINGS MIRACULOUS

The concept of Miracle Mornings was created by the author Hal Elrod with the premise that how you start your day largely determines the quality of your day, your work, and your life. The Miracle Morning gives you a morning ritual and offers tips on how to get up early in the morning and to frame the day is a positive way.

The steps are found in the acronym life **S.A.V.E.R.S.,** which encourages you to do the following:

▸ Silence: Using a time of silence for reflection or meditation

▸ Affirmation: Saying positive declarations or pronouncements

▸ Visualization: Forming the mental images of what you want to achieve in your life

▸ Read: Reading something positive, uplifting, inspirational, or motivational

▸ Exercise: Physical activity that increases your heart rate and improves your circulation

▸ Scribing: Writing or journaling

These practices encourage you to review your morning routine and start implementing effective strategies to achieve your best life. You may choose to use Hal's framework, or you can create your own Miracle Mornings.

38. PLAY THE GRATITUDE GAME

I am uncertain where I learned this game, and some days I believe I may have created it, but it has been a source of strength during times I have felt as though I wasn't enough or I didn't possess enough. This game asks that you go through the alphabet, starting with the letter A, and list at least five things for which you are thankful that start with that letter. You then move on to the next letter.

The last time I played this game, I was thankful for the delicious apples in my kitchen, the air conditioner hard at work keeping me cool, my Aunt Bev whom I adore and my Aunt Greta who is hilarious, my sweet Uncle Alfred who has since passed, and the wonderful lifestyle medicine conference I attended in Arizona. I would do this with each alphabet, and generally by the time I've reached the letter C, I become overwhelmed with gratitude and realized just how full my life is. This game forces you to see that our lives are more abundant than we realize, but sometimes we have to force ourselves to see it.

So go ahead and play the gratitude game!

39. GRATITUDE BEFORE AND AFTER BED

I have found that practicing gratitude before bed and first in the morning is the best way to end and begin my day, respectively. At nights, I use my journal to list three things that happened that day for which I was grateful. This practice, like the gratitude game, forces you to focus on the blessings of your life. When gratitude is practiced early in the morning, it allows you to frame your day with hope and the expectation of great things.

40. FIKA

Fika is literally interpreted as a coffee break and is a ritual practice in in Sweden. It is generally a time set aside for the gathering of family, friends, and colleagues so they may take a break from the busyness of life. Some people use fika for alone time. Fika could take place at a coffee shop or at home. Either way, it's a great opportunity to get away from the hustle and bustle of day-to-day living and allows you to reconnect with yourself or your loved ones. Best of all, you don't have to be in Sweden to practice fika. Fika anyone?

41. FRILUFSTIV

This practice comes to us from Norway and represents being present with nature. It involves the love and appreciation of the outdoors and can include activities such as walking in the park, fishing, playing in the snow, gardening, and biking. This practice does not need to include equipment. My favorite practice of being out in nature involves going for a brisk walk in Central Park in New York City. Not only do I get to enjoy the benefits of the exericse, but I also get inspiration from others who are also exercising. It allows me to connect with nature, reduce stress, increase creativity, improve vitamin D production, and marvel at the beauty of the trees and flowers. The Norwegians are on to something since a recent study showed that women who are surrounded by nature lived longer, healthier lives.

How will you practice frilufstiv?

42. PRACTICE OPTIMISM

The ebb and flow of life dictates that after the sun comes rain, after the day comes night, after birth come death, and after joy comes sorrow. One trick for dealing with the rhythm of life is to practice optimism and look for the lesson in every negative experience. Another strategy is to view the failure as the universe forcing you to grow and redirecting your path. Finally, avoid dwelling in the negative place for too long and remember that every pity party must have an expiration date.

43. SMILE

Smile even when you don't feel like it, and this may lift your mood. Psychologists have known for a long time that physical changes can trigger an emotional reaction, and genuine smiles are believed to have a powerful impact on your health. That said, even a forced outer smile may have a positive effect on your wellbeing. Not only is smiling good for you, but it is contagious and may positively change someone else's mood and health.

5 Benefits of a Smile:

▶ Improves your mood

▶ Relieves stress

▶ Lowers your blood pressure

▶ Releases feel-good hormones

▶ Improves your positivity

44. LAUGHTER IS THE BEST MEDICINE

Laughter is the big sister of smile, and she not only brings good health to the body, but she can calm the mind as well. Laughter offers a positive antidote for stress and anxiety and can encourage easier forgiveness. Studies have also shown that people who laugh more often outlive those who don't.

5 Benefits of Laughter:

▶ Boosts the immune system

▶ Relaxes the body

▶ Improves blood flow

▶ Reduces stress and anxiety

▶ Burns calories

45. GIVE SOMEONE A HUG

The act of embracing someone can improve the mood, communicate warm feelings, offer comfort, provide support, and help reduce stress. The importance of hugs is often seen during painful situations where almost instinctively the default gesture is a hug. Hugs are seen as a survival instinct, and it seems that the more hugs you give, the more positive the effect for both the hugger and huggee. The best part is that hugs are free.

46. PRACTICE THE PRINCIPLE OF UBUNTU

Ubuntu is a celebration of humanity towards others and is a philosophy that originated in South Africa with the Zulu tribe. Archbishop Desmond Tutu has been quoted with, "A person with ubuntu is open and available to others, affirming of others, does not feel threatened that others are able and good, for he or she has a proper self-assurance that comes from knowing that he or she belongs in a greater whole and is diminished when others are tortured or oppressed." He goes on to explain that ubuntu allows you to live to your highest potential and to see the potential in others. It also allows us to celebrate the wonder of our diversity and to be who we are. He explains it as "I am because we are."

47.   SAY NO TO NEGATIVITY

We all have that family member or friend who sees everything in a negative light. I have one such family member. If I say I plan on achieving a particular goal, she tells me all the reasons why I shouldn't pursue it, shows me why I will most certainly fail, and even have several people who have tried it and failed call me to talk me out of it. It took a few experiences with this person to notice the pattern, and initially I assumed the person wanted to limit my potential. I have now taken a different view and realize that most people give us advise based on the limitations they see for themselves. So, if that person assumes they would fail at the activity, they make the same conclusion about you. Often, their negativity is actually their way of trying to protect you.

I have found that the best way to handle these people is to first recognize the pattern, and consider sharing your goals with these people only after you have already accomplished them. And for the naysayers who simply want you to fail, remember that some people are meant to be loved from afar.

THINGS TO HELP ME TRANSFORM

_____

_____

_____

_____

_____

_____

_____

_____

_____

_____

_____

_____

_____

_____

_____

_____

THINGS TO HELP ME TRANSFORM

THINGS TO HELP ME TRANSFORM

THINGS TO HELP ME TRANSFORM

_____

_____

_____

_____

_____

_____

_____

_____

_____

_____

_____

_____

_____

_____

_____

CHAPTER 4

Nutrition

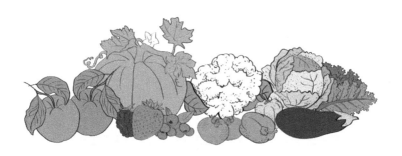

Eating well is a form of self-respect.
~**Unknown**

48. MINDFUL EATING

The practice of mindfulness encourages people to be present in the moment and to experience everything as it is happening. Mindfulness can be practiced with just about anything, including the way in which we consume food. In today's busy society, people often eat while multitasking. Since it takes about twenty minutes for the brain to realize that the stomach is full, mindless eating can lead to overeating. It also leaves very little room for meal enjoyment, increases the tendency to eat too quickly, encourages unhealthy food consumption, and may result in late-night eating or eating when you are not actually hungry.

10 Tips for Eating Mindfully:

▶ Before you begin eating, ask yourself, "Am I hungry?" If the answer is no, have a drink of water and move away from the food.

▶ Begin the meal with gratitude and pay attention to the color, shapes, and smell.

▶ Don't wait until you are ravenously hungry to eat.

▶ Eat your food from a small plate (nine inches or less).

▶ Take small bites.

▶ Eat slowly to allow your brain to catch up with the signals from your stomach.

▶ Don't rush through your meal. Give yourself 20 to 30 minutes to complete a meal.

▶ Chew your food for longer periods.

▶ Avoid eating while multitasking.

▶ Try using chopsticks, as you have a tendency to eat more slowly.

49. KNOW THYSELF

About 20 Christmases ago, my beloved Aunt Bev baked several Jamaican sweet potato puddings. She knew that sweet potato pudding, laden with artery-clogging butter and blood glucose-spiking sugar, is a favorite of mine. From a place of kindness and love, she gave me a pudding the size of a sheet cake. If I had to guess, the entire thing was easily 10,000 calories.

Pretty soon, I was having sweet potato pudding for breakfast, as a midmorning snack, after lunch, as a dessert after dinner, and with tea before bed. In five days, a pudding that could have easily served twenty people was finished.

While a few lucky souls can consistently eat unhealthy food in moderation, the vast majority of people can't limit themselves to just one spoon of ice cream, or my case, one slice of sweet potato pudding. If you know you are someone for whom willpower will fail, and that's the case for most people, avoid indulging in the unhealthy activity all together. By the way, I have never accepted an entire sweet potato pudding since then. I now know myself and understand my weaknesses.

50. STROKE-SMART EATING

Strokes result in tremendous disability and can significantly change your life and your ability to function. After many years of being the Medical Director of a stroke specialty acute in-patient rehabilitation unit, I know for sure that even the best rehabilitation is never as good as never having the stroke to begin with. Although several of the risk factors for stroke are beyond our control (age, race, family history), there are many lifestyle-related changes we can make to significantly reduce our risk of this deadly and disabling disorder. Nutrition can play a significant role in preventing a stroke and reducing the risk of recurrence. One smart approach is to view eating with the knowledge that food is medicine, and the things you put in your mouth can either heal or harm.

13 Strategies for Stroke-Smart Eating:

▸ Eat five to seven servings of fruits and vegetables on a daily basis.

▸ Focus on a whole food plant-based diet.

▶ Follow the "Healthy Plate" by ensuring at least half of each plate consist of fruits and veggies.

▶ Select a rainbow of colors for the fruits and vegetables to increase the variety of nutrients.

▶ Avoid refined sugar.

▶ Choose whole grains over processed white rice or flour.

▶ Keep your salt intake to less than 2,400 milligrams per day.

▶ Recognize that sea salt is salt and will have the same effect on your blood pressure.

▶ Limit your alcohol intake.

▶ Limit your intake of saturated fat and trans fat.

▶ Get your nutrients from foods and not from supplements.

▶ Avoid over-consuming foods and pay attention to portion sizes.

▶ Increase your fiber intake.

51.   COOK YOUR OWN FOOD

A few weeks ago, I watched a video where a cook at a famous restaurant shared the secret recipe for their award-winning fried chicken. The secret involved soaking the chicken over-night in salted water, followed by battering and deep frying the following day. I listened to her and learned that a person with high blood pressure could have ordered that chicken without realizing that it had been soaked in salted water, and this could have resulted in a spike in blood pressure.

Cooking your own food allows you to choose the freshest and best ingredients and prevents you from being exposed to salts and sugar that are often added by restaurants. Cooking at home also gives you the opportunity to improve your cooking skills, allows you to save money and time, and facilitates connection with your loved ones.

If you are not a good cook, you can borrow cook books, join a class, watch videos on YouTube, swap recipes, or join an online healthy cooking group. Can't find a group? Consider creating one yourself.

5 Healthy Cookbooks:

▶ *The How Not to Die Cookbook* by Michael Greger, MD

▶ *Forks Over Knives: The Cookbook* by Del Sroufe

▶ *The Prevent and Reverse Heart Disease Cookbook* by Ann Crile Esselstyn and Jane Esselstyn

▶ *The Healthiest Diet on the Planet* by John McDougall, MD

▶ *Healthy Vegan* by Nicole Beckford

52.   MAINTAIN A FOOD DIARY

Food diaries are often used by physicians, dieticians, health coaches, and other health providers to help document not only what is consumed, but also the quantity eaten, the preparation of the food, and the time of day the food was consumed. Information deducted from this includes whether or not you are eating mindlessly, having trouble with portion control, eating when you are emotionally stressed, or eating unhealthy foods. Often, if we are to verbally identify what we eat, we tend to under-report. It is not unusual for an overweight patient to say, "I am not sure why I am gaining weight because I really don't eat much." Evaluation via a food diary helps to highlight the frequency of unhealthy snacks, liquid calories in the form of sodas and juices, and the actual quantity of food consumed.

Food diaries allow for awareness and provide the opportunities for improvement. Studies have shown that keeping a food diary is an important key to sustainable weight loss.

53.   THE PRINCIPLE OF HARA HACHI BU

Okinawan are one of the groups that make up the Blue Zones—the five regions in the world where people live longer, healthier lives than average. At the time of the writing of this book, the Okinawan population is said to be about one million, and of those, about 900 are centenarians. This number is about four times higher than the average in America or Britain.

In studies of this population, it has been found that not only do the types of food they eat seem to play a role in their longevity, but also the quantity of the food they consume. Most Okinawans eat from small plates and practice the Japanese principle of Hara Hachi Bu, which is a traditional teaching that instructs people to eat until they are only 80 percent full.

Eating until you are 80 percent full encourages you to eat until you are satisfied and decreases your chance of overeating.

54. ELIMINATE PROCESSED FOODS

Processed foods are generally associated a low nutritional value, higher calorie count, and added sugars, fats, and unhealthy chemicals. In general, a processed food is any food that has undergone a deliberate change prior to it being consumed. They are easily identified on supermarket shelves in boxes, bags, or packages. Foods that are highly processed are also generally cheap, fast, and can often be found in a vending machine.

Try to minimize process foods and have a goal of completely eliminating them from your diet.

10 Tips to Help You Eliminate Processed Foods:

▶ Surround yourself with healthy foods such as fruits and vegetables.

▶ Avoid anything in boxes, bags, or cans.

▶ Have healthy snacks available.

▶ Learn to read food labels.

▶ Avoid foods with more than four ingredients listed.

▶ Visit your local farmer's market on a regular basis.

▶ Get a garden and grow your own vegetables.

▶ Learn to cook.

▶ Pack leftover foods that you cooked for lunch.

▶ Avoid fast food restaurants.

55. WHOLE FOOD PLANT-BASED DIET

It's no secret that plants in the form of fruits and vegetables are powerful in our diet and are known to prevent, stop, and even reverse some of our deadliest diseases. Yet only about one in ten Americans consume enough fruits and vegetables. The current Standard American Diet is indeed SAD. It is known to contribute to numerous chronic diseases and leaves little room for the five to seven servings of fruits and vegetables that will protect us against most lifestyle diseases. Plants are powerful and contain proteins, vitamins, and minerals.

The whole food plant-based (WFPB) way of eating is a dietary pattern that focuses on fruits, vegetable, and whole grains. It also includes legumes, nuts, and seeds in moderation. This way of eating is seen as one the most effective ways to fight diseases, reduce obesity, and improve your wellness. It discourages meat (including poultry and fish), eggs, dairy, sugar, oils, or processed foods. It recommends eating foods as close to their natural state as possible (e.g. an apple instead of apple juice or the sweet potato instead of sweet potato pies).

The WFPB diet is different from veganism in that, although the latter excludes all animal products, a diet high in processed foods such as potato chips or pastries could still be considered vegan but would not qualify as WFPB.

10 Strategies for Success with the Whole Food Plant-Based Diet:

▸ Evaluate your refrigerator and pantry and begin to swap out processed foods, which are often found in boxes and bags.

▸ Don't drink your calories in the form of sodas or juices. Have water or seltzer instead.

▸ Consume more beans, lentils, and peas.

▸ Make a commitment to eat vegetables at every meal.

▸ Fill half your plate with vegetables and fruits.

▸ If you eat meat every day, begin to decrease the frequency with meatless Mondays.

▸ Add a vegetarian option to your holiday meals.

▸ Begin to eliminate red meat, fish, poultry, eggs, and deli meats from your diet.

▸ If you eat fish, limit to twice per week to reduce your risk of mercury poisoning.

▸ Eat whole grains and avoid processed foods such as white breads, pastries, and cookies.

56. THE HEALTHY PLATE

The Healthy Eating Plate, created by nutrition experts at Harvard School of Public Health and editors at Harvard Health Publications, provides detailed guidance to help you make the best eating choices. The Healthy Plate may be used with any meal, during any occasion, and across ethnicities.

It uses a nine-inch round plate, and an imaginary line is created to divide the plate in half. One half should be mostly vegetables, and a smaller portion of it may include fruits. The other half will be divided into two halves, with one half containing healthy proteins and the other half consisting of whole grains.

The trick with proteins is to choose healthy ones. For example, luncheon meats, hot dogs, and bacon are proteins, but they are also highly processed with high sodium content. On the other hand, beans, legumes, and vegetables provide high-quality proteins.

It is also important that you choose healthy options in the whole grain section. To do this, avoid all white bread, white rice, cold breakfast cereals, quick-cook oat, and pastries. Instead, opt for steel-cook oatmeal, flaxseed, quinoa, and brown rice.

57. SHOP IN THE PRODUCE AISLE FIRST

Previously, consumers were encouraged to shop around the perimeter of the grocery store because many stores tended to stock more of the healthier items around the perimeter. Today, though, foods on the other end include cheeses and other dairy products, processed meats, and baked goods. The best advice then is to make a beeline for the produce aisle and spend the majority of your time and money there. Better yet, find an inexpensive farmer's market where your food is more likely to be fresh and may contain fewer pesticides.

58. UNDERSTAND THE FOOD LABEL

Understanding the food label is one way to ensure you understand how much and what you are putting in your body. A healthy diet is one that contains many fruits and vegetables, which generally doesn't contain food labels. If you chose foods with labels, you should understand the major items on the labels. Another thing to consider is that details about the protein in your food are not required to be on the label. It is important to choose more plants for your protein source. And yes, plants have protein. If you don't believe, remember that the cows you eat for your source of protein get theirs from plants. Why are you eating the middle man?

10 Things to Look at on a Food Label:

▶ Start with the serving size as this will tell you the number of servings in the container.

▶ Look to see how many calories are in each serving.

▶ Look at the percent daily values to see what percent of a 2,000-calorie diet the serving represents.

▶ Look at specific values such as the cholesterol, fats, sodium, and fiber.

▶ Understand what the quantity means. For example, low sodium is 140 milligrams of sodium or less per serving.

▶ When the label says calorie free, it means there are less than five calories per serving.

▶ Fat free or sugar free should contain less than half a gram of fat or sugar per serving.

▶ Cholesterol free means the food must contain fewer than two milligrams of cholesterol and two grams or less of saturated fat per serving.

▶ Look to see if the food gives a source of vitamins or minerals.

▶ Focus on high-fiber foods.

59. THE WATER SAUTÉ

Once simple way to cut out oil in general and heated oil in particular is to prepare your vegetables using water sauté. Instead of using oil to stir fry vegetables, try using vegetable broth or water. Since your taste buds and your brain have grown accustomed to the taste of the fat from the oil, the first couple of times eating this way may require some adjustments. If allowed, however, both your brain and taste buds will adjust.

5 Steps of the Water Sauté:

▶ Add about six tablespoons of water or vegetable broth to pan and put on medium heat.

▶ Allow the water or vegetable broth to begin steaming in the pan.

▶ Add diced onions, scallion, tomatoes, green peppers, minced garlic, and powdered seasoning.

▶ Stir, then add in chopped vegetables.

▶ Lower heat and cover. Stir to prevent sticking and add additional liquid as needed.

Turn off the stove and enjoy!

60.   INCREASE INTAKE OF FRUITS AND VEGETABLES

Michael Pollan is credited with the quote: "Eat foods, not too much, mostly plants." The current recommendations for fruits and vegetables encourage that we eat at least five to seven per servings day. Even with good evidence of the benefits of this eating pattern, most Americans manage to achieve much less than this.

5 Strategies to Increase Intake of Fruits and Vegetables:

▸   Ensure that your refrigerator has enough of the vegetables and fruits you enjoy.

▸   Cook your own meals containing a large number of vegetables and pack leftovers for lunch.

▸   Pack a fruit for lunch and for travel.

▸   When eating out, preview the menu ahead of time to ensure there are vegetarian options.

▸   Reimagine breakfast. Ditch the typical breakfast food and have a bowl of water-sautéed kale.

61.   BRING YOUR LIFESTYLE WITH YOU

I recently went to couple of medical conferences, and after a week of travel and hotel living, I gained a few pounds. Between the airport food, hotel snacks, concierge lounge, and unhealthy conference foods, I found myself in a similar boat as some of my coaching clients. I learned that to continue my healthy lifestyle, I needed to do a better job of planning for my travel and bring my lifestyle with me. You can do the same.

10 Tips for Healthier Travel:

▶ Have a plan. In the same way you pack and plan excursions, have an eating plan for travel.

▶ Track what you eat in your journal.

▶ Take healthy snacks with you on the plane and break that out while everyone else is having cookies.

▶ Ensure you drink enough water to adequately hydrate yourself.

▶ Some hotels have a mini fridge. Go to the grocery store and stock up on healthy foods.

▶ The gyms at many hotels tend to have a ready supply of fresh fruits.

▶ Use an online search engine to find healthy options.

▶ Consider hotels with a kitchen area to allow for cooking.

▶ Ensure that you stick to your dietary restrictions even while you are on the road.

▶ Avoid late-night eating.

62.   EAT LIGHT AT NIGHT

There is a popular saying that admonishes us to "eat breakfast like a king, lunch like a prince, and dinner like a pauper." Current research seems to have caught up with this sage advice and it now appears that not only what you eat matters, but also when you eat it. Also, our bodies seem to process food differently if we eat and then go for a brisk walk versus eating and then going to bed. Heavy eating at night can exacerbate reflux and result in indigestion, negatively impact sleep, and lead to weight gain and obesity.

63.   THE SECRET WEAPON OF MEAL PREPPING

One of the best strategies to help save time and money and also ensure healthier eating is meal prepping. In a well-executed meal preparation, I block several hours on a Sunday to cook two different meals and package them into small single-serving containers. I generally keep only two days' worth in the refrigerator, and the rest is frozen and then thawed as needed.

I eat what I make, so I know the exact ingredients and I save money and time. Pre-packing the meals also ensures I eat the correct serving size.

Make meal prepping fun by including your family.

64.   THE POWER OF PORTION CONTROL

The portion, or the amount of food consumed, is an individual choice and can make or break your weight management plan. Consuming too much food, especially with no physical activity, can lead to weight gain and obesity. Even when eating healthy foods, if you eat the amount for two people, you can pack on the pounds. When you read food labels, you will know exactly how much of the food item represents a serving size. Another quick and dirty way to get an estimation of the serving size is to use a hand-based portion size.

Hand-Based Portion Size:

▶ With a hand-based portion size, a fist represents a cup. This is best used for a serving of fruits, vegetables, rice, and pasta.

▶ The palm represents about a three-ounce serving. This is best used for meat, fish, and poultry.

▶ Two handfuls represent an ounce of chips, pretzels, or popcorn.

▶ A handful represents an ounce of nuts or raisins.

▶ A thumb represents an ounce of hard cheese, almond butter, or peanut butter.

▸ The tip of the thumb represents a teaspoon of sugar, cooking oil, butter, or mayonnaise.

65. GREEN LEAFY VEGETABLES ARE A GIFT

Green leafy vegetables are a great source of nutrition. They are high in vitamins such as A, C, E, and K and are rich in the antioxidant carotenoids. Vegetables such as bok choy and broccoli are also high in the B vitamins. Vegetables in general are high in fiber, iron, magnesium, potassium, and calcium, and they are filling yet low in calories. Vegetables have been credited with helping with illness prevention, and in some cases, disease reversal. Populations with diets high in vegetables tend to avoid some of the chronic or lifestyle diseases often seen in people who eat a standard American diet or SAD diet.

Since we know vegetables are integral to good health, our primary goal should be finding ways to increase our intake of these vegetables in our lives.

5 Strategies to Increase Vegetable Intake:

▸ Reimagine breakfast and have a warm bowl of water-sautéed green leafy vegetables.

▸ Take a salad for lunch.

▸ Have a vegetable smoothie.

▶ Check out cookbooks or YouTube for recipes with green leafy vegetables.

▶ Experiment with vegetables you know little about.

66. BEANS ARE YOUR BUDDIES

Beans represent one of the most inexpensive sources of fiber and protein. The consumption of beans seems to be a common practice among the healthiest groups of people in the world. Beans can be used as an entire meal, the main entree, or as a side dish. They are also very versatile and may be used in soups, stews, and casseroles and partnered with brown rice or potatoes.

What's not often recognized about beans is that that they are an excellent source of nutrients and are one of your best ammunitions in protecting your health and preventing disease.

10 Health Benefits of Beans:

▶ Help stabilize blood sugar and prevent diabetes

▶ High in folate, which is known to help prevent neural tube defects during pregnancy

▶ High in a type of antioxidant called polyphenol, which helps to fight free radicals

▶ Associated with a reduction in heart diseases and stroke

- Prevent cancers such as colon cancer

- Help to prevent obesity due to their low calorie count, nutrient density, and high fiber, which keeps you feeling full

- Curb the appetite and help to prevent overeating

- Reduce the aging process

- Decrease inflammation

- Prevent fatty liver disease

10 of My Favorite Beans:

- Kidney beans

- Lima beans

- Pigeon peas

- Black beans

- Navy beans

- Pinto beans

- Garbanzo beans

- Red beans

- Soy beans

- Black-eyed peas

67. THE VICIOUS SUGAR CYCLE

The sugar cycle is a balance between various hormones in the body including leptin (the appetite suppressor that keeps you lean) and ghrelin (the greedy gremlin that keeps you hungry). When you eat high amounts of processed foods, the sugar levels spike, resulting in the pancreas releasing insulin to address the sugar surge. Upon release, the function of insulin is to rid the blood stream of sugar in order to regain homeostasis or balance. If, however, too much insulin is released, the blood sugar may drop too low, resulting in you feeling hungry and again eating to deal with the low blood sugar. Insulin functions like an anabolic hormone and encourages the body to store fat. The cycle keeps repeating with risk of weight gain and poor health unless the individual changes the types of food they consume.

To hijack the sugar cycle, reach for foods that are high in fiber and of low glycemic index. Foods such as beans, fruits, vegetables, whole grains, and flaxseeds are high in fiber and help stave off the sudden rise in blood sugar. Avoid sugary beverages, pastries, and other processed foods.

68. FIBER IS YOUR FRIEND

Fiber is a very important part of a healthy nutrition. Fiber-rich foods tend to be low in calories, and fruits and vegetables are high in fiber and healthy nutrients. Fiber also helps with feeling full, thereby decreasing the risk of overeating, and may decrease the risk of weight gain and obesity. Fiber also helps to move waste product quickly through the gastrointestinal track, prevents constipation, and decrease prolonged exposure to toxins. It has also been found that a high-fiber diet may decrease the risk of certain types of cancers such as colon cancer. The general recommendation is to consume 25-40 grams per day of fiber.

15 Fiber-Rich Foods to Include in Your Diet:

▶ Chia seeds

▶ Flax seeds

▶ Popcorn

▶ Almonds

▶ Oats

▶ Artichoke

▶ Chickpeas

▶ Lentils

▶ Kidney beans

▶ Split peas

▶ Avocado

▶ Pears

▶ Apples

▶ Strawberries

▶ Bran flakes

69. THE HEALTH BENEFITS OF KEEPING HYDRATED

Most people are already dehydrated by the time they experience thirst. The cells in your body need water to function. When the cells are dehydrated, the body begins to extract water from the blood stream leading to dehydration. Extra perspiration may also contribute to further water loss. Evidence of this dehydration may be noticed in your dark-colored urine.

In order to decrease the risk of dehydration, keep track of the amount of fluids you take in on a daily basis, hydrate with water and avoid sugary beverages, and eat plenty of fruits and vegetables, which naturally contain water. Also, be aware that certain fluids such as caffeinated beverages and beers tend to have a diuretic effect and may result in water loss and further the dehydration.

5 Ways to Increase Water Intake:

▶ Keep a full bottle of water on your desk at all times

▶ Use a water reminder app

▶ Track your water intake with an app or use your food diary

▶ Carbonated water and decaffeinated herbal tea also count towards your water intake

▶ Try infused water or iced teas

70. INTERMITTENT FASTING

Intermittent fasting represents an eating style in which you eat within a specific window and the rest of the time you don't eat, also known as the fasting window. Practitioners of this way of eating don't generally see this as a diet and instead it is viewed as a lifestyle. There are several variations of this way of eating. Below is a list of some forms of intermittent fasting. Since fasting can seriously affect certain diseases, it is important that you speak with your doctor prior to attempting any types of fasting.

There has been some research that suggest a relationship between skipping breakfast and weight gain but the relationship does not appear to be a causative one. The research suggests that when people skip breakfast, they tend to overeat processed foods and unhealthy foods to make up for the hunger. Others have skipped breakfast and have done well. The best suggestion is to see what works best for you and have a discussion with your physician before starting any plan.

7 Popular Ways to do Intermittent Fasting:

▸ Fast-Five: You eat in a five-hour window and fast for the other 19 hours.

▸ Fast-Eight: You eat in an eight-hour window and fast for the other 16 hours.

▸ 5:2 Diet: Eat healthy and regularly for five days per week, restricting calories to 500 for women or 600 for men or fast for two days per week.

▸ Every other day: Also known as the alternate day fast, allows eating one day followed by fasting the next.

▸ OMAD: One meal a day

▸ Eat-Stop-Eat: The person fasts for a 24-hour period once or twice per week.

▸ Bulletproof Intermittent Fasting: The individual skips breakfast and has Bulletproof Coffee instead. Bulletproof coffee, also known as keto coffee, refers to coffee with a high amount of fats and is often a combination of coffee, butter, coconut oil, and medium chain triglyceride (MCT) oil.

71.   MIRACLE MORINGA

Moringa Olifera is a plant native to India but grows in Africa, Asia, the Caribbean, and South America and is often called the miracle tree or the drumstick plant. It has been used for centuries to help with malnutrition and for its antifungal, antiviral, anti-diabetes, and anti-inflammatory properties. Moringa has been shown to contain proteins, minerals, and vitamins and is believed to have very few side effects. The oil from Moringa is used for hair growth, to maintain youthful looking skin, and to treat rashes. It is said to be low in fats and contains no cholesterol. Moringa has been widely researched in America, and in parts of Africa there have been experiments looking at the benefits of Moringa on sickle cell anemia.

13 Nutrients Found in Moringa:

▶ Vitamin A

▶ Vitamin B1 (thiamine)

▶ Vitamin B2 (riboflavin)

▶ Vitamin B3 (niacin)

▶ Vitamin B6

▶ Folate

▶ Ascorbic Acid (Vitamin C)

▶ Calcium

▶ Potassium

▶ Iron

- ▶ Phosphorus

- ▶ Magnesium

- ▶ Zinc

72. CURCUMIN

This orange root related to the ginger family has been used in India for many years and is the spice that gives curry its yellow color. Aside from its use in foods, it is popularly used as a medicinal herb and supplement.

Curcumin is said to be a strong antioxidant and is the main active ingredient in turmeric. It is believed that curcumin is best absorbed in the presence of black pepper, which tends to be added to most supplements. It is also said to be fat soluble and is therefore better absorbed with a fatty meal. Care should be taken if you are on blood thinners since curcumin is thought to have blood thinning properties. As with any supplements, clearance should be sought by your doctor prior to initiating.

10 Reported Benefits of Curcumin:

- ▶ Natural anti-inflammatory compound

- ▶ May improve the symptoms of arthritis

- ▶ May have anti-aging properties

- Increases the antioxidant capacity of the body

- May lower the risk of heart disease

- May have anti-cancer properties

- Appears to boost brain-derived neurotrophic factor, linked to improved brain function

- May have a role in Alzheimer's prevention or treatment

- May help to improve the mood

- May have blood thinning properties

THINGS TO HELP ME TRANSFORM

_____

_____

_____

_____

_____

_____

_____

_____

_____

_____

_____

_____

_____

_____

_____

_____

THINGS TO HELP ME TRANSFORM

THINGS TO HELP ME TRANSFORM

_____

_____

_____

_____

_____

_____

_____

_____

_____

_____

_____

_____

_____

_____

_____

_____

THINGS TO HELP ME TRANSFORM

CHAPTER 5

Self-Care

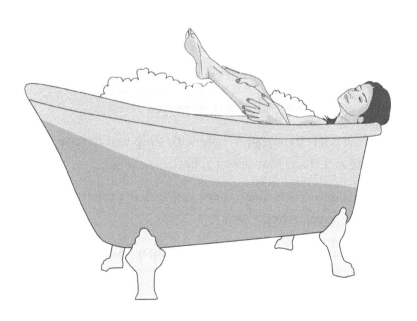

*If your compassion does not include
yourself, it is incomplete.*

~Jack Kornfield

73. AROMATHERAPY

Aromatherapy is a form of therapy that uses essential oils. These aromatic essential oils are extracted from plants and are believed to penetrate through the skin and into the olfactory system. It is believed that the oils can improve mood, lower blood pressure, relieve muscle tension, decrease pulse rate, reduce pain, and improve cerebral function. There is the risk of allergic reaction and skin sensitivity if oils are applied directly to the skin. Since it is not known how essential oils may interact with certain medications or whether or not it could cause issues during pregnancy, get clearance from your doctor before adding it to your regimen.

10 Essential Oils and Their Reported Uses:

▸ Lavender: Reported to help with sleep and to have calming and stress reduction properties

▸ Rosemary: Believed to have anti-cancer properties and to play a role in brain health

▸ Grapefruit: Said to help ease hangovers, decrease sugar cravings, and calm anxiety

- Eucalyptus: Believed to help reduce fever, relieve respiratory disorders, and improve brain health

- Geranium: Said to help with premenstrual tension and cramps

- Peppermint: May help relieve joint pain, cool hot flashes, energize, and promote hair growth

- Orange: Believed to help relieve respiratory infection and to promote youthful skin

- Tea Tree: Used for various skin conditions and said to be a bug repellant

- Frankincense: Said to help calm the mind and promote awareness

- Clove: Used for tooth ache and dental abscess; said to have antifungal properties

74. DRY BRUSHING

This self-care procedure involves the brushing of the skin with a stiff dry brush. It is known to help with exfoliation and increase blood flow. Although the evidence to back up its use is scant, those who practice dry brushing believe it improves circulation and helps with digestion. When done consistently, it may help reduce the appearance of cellulite. It is recommended to brush in the direction of lymph flow. If you choose to practice this form of self-care, remember that the brushes used tend to have firm bristles, so care should be taken if you are on blood thinners, if you have thin skin, or if the integrity of your skin is compromised with cuts or rashes.

75. PLANT PLANTS

Plants, believed to offer physical and psychological benefits and stress reduction, may be an overlooked way of promoting wellbeing. Plants have the power to improve the esthetics of a place and may improve mood and reduce stress. Even deeper than that, plants can help to absorb sounds, and some plants are known to release oxygen and help to improve air quality.

5 Plants Known to Help with Air Quality:

▸ Snake Plant: Believed to remove trichlorobenzene, formaldehyde, xylene, and benzene

▸ Garden Mum: Said to help with removal of ammonia, benzene, formaldehyde, and xylene

▸ Spider Plant: Believed to help with removal of formaldehyde and xylene

▸ Peace Lilly: Reportedly removes formaldehyde, trichloroethylene, ammonia, and benzene

▸ Aloe Vera: Said to remove formaldehyde

76.   STEAM ROOM

A steam room is a room heated with moisture often used for relaxation, the burning of calories, post-workout stiffness, skin health, and sinus decongestion. In some practices, steam is used as a part of medical therapy. People who frequent steam rooms believe they help to improve circulation by dilating blood vessels, thereby improving blood and oxygen flow to tissues. The dilation of blood vessels may also result in blood pressure changes, so people with low or high blood pressure should seek clearance from their doctors before participating in this treatment. Since significant sweating is produced with steam room therapy, be sure to drink plenty of water before and after.

77.   SAUNAS

The use of heat therapy for healing dates back thousands of years with the belief that heat therapy offered detox for the body. Saunas produce dry heat and may induce considerable sweating. Today, there are various types of saunas, including traditional dry, steam, and infrared. Infrared saunas are further broken down into near, far, and full spectrum infrared.

Some supporters of sauna use believe that saunas mimic cardiovascular exercise due to the high heat, sweating, and increased blood flow. The current evidence supports the belief that saunas provide relaxation and stress reduction for many. Due to the vasodilation and possible impact on blood pressure, you should get clearance from your doctor before initiating this treatment.

78. CRYOTHERAPY

Cryotherapy is a new therapy with limited outcome studies and involves the use of freezing or near freezing temperatures. People practice cryotherapy in various ways from cold rooms to ice baths, but the most common practice is by sitting in a cryotherapy chamber for about five minutes. Because of the cold, some may find this therapy unpleasant.

The most common reasons for which people use cryotherapy include the reduction of inflammation and pain, weight loss, and anxiety management.

79. BODY SCRUBS

Body scrubs often use abrasive compounds to help remove dead cells. Other terms used include exfoliation, body polishing, and body gloss. Aside from the benefits of the appearance of smoother, revitalized, and more youthful looking skin, body scrubs have also been credited with inducing relaxation, improving circulation, and leaving the skin feeling more hydrated.

Because of the abrasive quality of body scrubs, care should be taken to avoid sensitive skin that has been compromised. Scrubs should also be avoided by people on medications with the active ingredient of retinol or any types of chemical exfoliants or peels or anticoagulants.

80. EAR CANDLING

Ear candling is a treatment in which a hollow candle is used for about ten to fifteen minutes. The practitioner places the pointed end of the candle in the client's ear and the slightly wider end is left outside of the ear and is lit. Practitioners of ear candling believe that the warmth created by the flame creates a suction action, which then pulls impurities from the ear.

There are no research trials showing that this works, but proponents of ear candling report relief or reduction of ear wax build up, tinnitus, ear ache, swimmer's ear, hearing problems, upper respiratory infection, vertigo, and stress. However, there have also been reports of the wax from candles building up in the ear after this procedure.

THINGS TO HELP ME TRANSFORM

_____

_____

_____

_____

_____

_____

_____

_____

_____

_____

_____

_____

_____

_____

_____

_____

_____

THINGS TO HELP ME TRANSFORM

THINGS TO HELP ME TRANSFORM

THINGS TO HELP ME TRANSFORM

CHAPTER 6

Faith and Spirituality

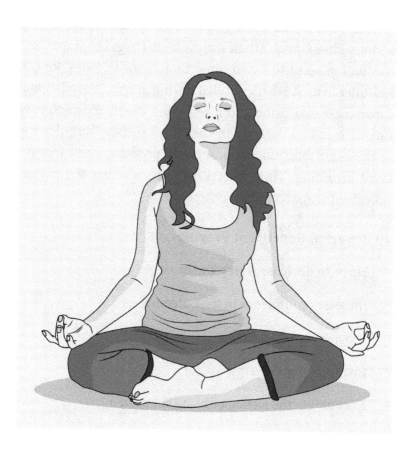

Just as a candle cannot burn without fire,
man cannot live without a spiritual life.

~**Buddha**

81. PRAYER

Praying is a personal experience for each individual, and although we don't yet understand scientifically how prayer works, we know that a large percent of people experiencing serious illness pray. Studies suggest that regular prayer and meditation seem to be an important factor in living longer, healthier lives. It is believed that during prayer, the individual experiences relaxation and a reduction in stress, which may further lead to a decrease in the body's metabolism, slowing of the heart rate, reduction of blood pressure, and more relaxed breathing. These effects are seen whether the person prays for themselves or for others.

10 Reported Benefits of Praying:

▶ Helps to decrease worry and anxiety

▶ Increases confidence in the outcome

▶ Provides encouragement

▶ Instills positive energy

▶ Encourages the feeling of being supported

▶ Increases the feeling of being connected to a higher power

▶ Helps with being more open to forgiveness

▶ Decreases judgement

▶ Helps adopt an attitude of gratitude

▶ Helps to improve focus

82. CRYSTAL HEALING

Crystal healing is a popular practice in health spas, new age clinics, and yoga studios. The belief is that crystals act as a conduit for healing by allowing positive energy to flow into the body, resulting in negative energy and diseases flowing out.

In crystal healing, it is believed that certain stones carry specific properties, and the practitioner places the stones or crystals on the body in certain designated points, often based on the disease or the location of the complaint. This healing can also take the form of wearing these stones or crystals on the body or placing them under the pillow to ward off negative energy or sickness.

Although there are no scientific studies showing its efficacy, there have been documented symptom improvements with the use of crystal therapy, some of which are believed to be related to placebo effect.

The Assigned Healing Properties of 5 Crystals:

▶ Green Aventurine: Helps the heart

▶ Amethyst: Beneficial for the intestine

▶ Yellow Topaz: Provides mental clarity

▶ Rose Quartz: Cultivates love

▶ Celestite: Relives stress

83. HARMONYUM

Hormonyum is a healing system initially developed to assist with self-healing. This practice is said to address diseases at an emotional and mental level with the goal that the disease does not manifest physically. The practice uses a predesigned set of movements where the practitioner minimally touches the recipient, and the goal is to achieve a state of deep relaxation and restoration of a state of balance and harmony.

My exposure to Hormonyum came at a Naam Yoga studio where I enjoyed treatments in exchange for money I had paid for teacher training. I had eight sessions of Harmonyum, and while I can't say it changed anything specific about my health, I will say it helped induce a state of relaxation.

84. MUDRA

Mudras are a combination of subtle physical movements that are said to alter mood, attitude, and perception and to deepen awareness and concentration. Mudras may involve the whole body in conjunction with yoga poses, breathing techniques, or visualization techniques, or they be a simple hand position. It is believed that each mudra sets up a different link and has corresponding effect on the body or mind. The practitioners of mudra believe that disease is imbalance in the body, and mudras are able to adjust the flow of energy and help facilitate healing and restore health.

85. FORGIVENESS

Many years ago, while still a teen, I felt a close family friend had done me wrong. Over the years, when I'd think of her, I would boil with anger. Many years later, I saw the offender and she had her arms wide open to embrace. I realized that I had spent years in anger, and she had long forgotten about the event.

Forgiveness involves a decision to let go of resentment and any thoughts of revenge. It doesn't mean that you don't acknowledge your hurt or that the person is excused from their action. It does mean that don't allow yourself to be held prisoner to the other person's action, and if you allow your-self, you may even understand why that person acted in the manner they did. Most of the time, their actions are not even about you.

5 Tips to Help you Forgive:

▶ Know that it's okay to acknowledge that you were hurt.

▶ Make the decision to forgive.

▶ Understand that forgiving the person helps you more than it helps them.

▶ Take the step to empathize or understand why the person may have taken the action.

▶ Look for the lesson.

THINGS TO HELP ME TRANSFORM

_____

_____

_____

_____

_____

_____

_____

_____

_____

_____

_____

_____

_____

_____

_____

_____

THINGS TO HELP ME TRANSFORM

_____

_____

_____

_____

_____

_____

_____

_____

_____

_____

_____

_____

_____

_____

_____

_____

THINGS TO HELP ME TRANSFORM

THINGS TO HELP ME TRANSFORM

CHAPTER 7

Optimize Brain Health

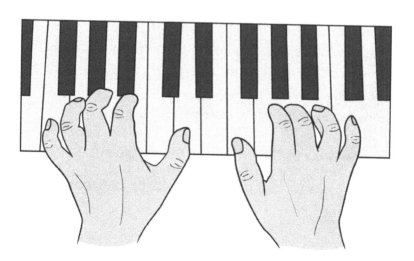

Brain disease starts in your daily bread.
                              ~**Dr. David Perlmutter**

86. STAY MENTALLY AND PHYSICALLY ACTIVE

The benefits of physical activity and exercise on the brain are well documented. We now know from research that brain-derived neurotrophic factor (BDNF), a protein produced by the brain that has been described as "Miracle-Gro" for the brain, is increased with exercise. We also know that exercise can increase the number of brain cells and that the hippocampus—the part of the brain known to be involved with memory and learning—increases in volume with exercise. What many people don't realize is that some research suggests that mental stimulation may also be good for the brain.

Some of our current research suggests that keeping the mind active seems to help sharpen the brain and stave off memory issues, which also translates to improved performance of daily tasks. Once a person has a diagnosis of Alzheimer's, mental exercises don't seem to reverse the cognitive impairment, so prevention seems to be the key.

10 Activities to Help Keep the Brain Sharp:

▶ Take a dance class that requires learning new steps or choreography.

▶ Learn a new language.

▶ Learn to play a new musical instrument.

▶ Work on crossword puzzles.

▶ Play online memory games.

▶ Take a writing class.

▶ Try Rubik's cube.

▶ Play Sudoku.

▶ Attend a lecture.

▶ Read books from various genres.

87. MEDITATION

Meditation uses the power of focus, redirects your thoughts, and helps you connect to your inner self. Meditation is now more mainstream, and there are studies to support the reports from practitioners that it improves self-awareness, relaxation, focus, mental clarity, happiness, pain, blood pressure, stress, and anxiety. In fact, there are studies that suggest that meditation also changes the brain by enhancing the sections involved with positive emotion and self-regulation.

The two main types of meditation are focused attention and open monitoring meditation. With focused attention, the practitioner focuses on a single a sound, thought, object, or visualization. Open monitoring, allows the practitioner to be aware of all aspects of the environment.

To try meditation, there are many free apps, videos on You Tube, podcasts, and centers that can aide with guided meditation.

88. GUIDED IMAGERY

The mind is very powerful and may be influenced by suggestion. Guided imagery is a form of meditation in which the practitioner follows the guidance of someone who aims to point them away from stress, pain, and anxiety with the use of words and images. It is believed to have some of the same benefits of meditation, such as reduction of stress and anxiety and improved blood pressure and sleep.

This practice is often used by elite athletes, who visualize themselves performing at their best, and studies suggest it helps their performance.

89. TEA TIME

Teas have been used by many cultures over the years, and they appear to be beneficial to health and wellness. The caffeine level of most teas is less than that of coffee, and some teas have disease-fighting antioxidants. Some studies on teas have suggested protection from cancer and heart disease, decreased cholesterol levels, weight loss, and decreased anxiety levels. The caffeinated varieties have the benefits of increased alertness and reduced fatigue. However, if caffeinated teas are consumed too late in the day, your sleep can be negatively affected. Teas are also versatile, as they may be consumed warm or cold. Some of the latest research suggests that having milk in black tea decreases the amounts of absorbed antioxidants. This seems to be the case for both cow's milk and soy milk.

10 Teas That Are Good for You:

▶ White: Believed to have potent anti-cancer properties

▶ Green: Least processed, highest in antioxidants, said to curb appetite

▶ Black: Abundant in antioxidants such as flavonoids, believed to help with heart disease

▶ Sage: Said to help with digestive problems and reduce the overproduction of perspiration

▶ Hibiscus: Lowers blood pressure

▶ Chamomile: Helps prevent complications from diabetes, known to induce relaxation

▶ Oolong: Shown to reduce bad cholesterol levels

▶ Pu-erh: A black tea shown to help with weight loss and reduction of cholesterol levels

▶ Rooibos: A red tea believed to have cancer-fighting properties

▶ Ginger: Believed to relieve nausea and motion sickness

90. THE BENEFITS OF BERRIES

It is no secret that berries are filled with nutrients such as polyphenols. It is believed that polyphenols may increase levels of nitric oxide, which is known to help relax blood vessels. Health benefits have been seen in good cholesterol levels, blood pressure, heart health, bone density, and cognitive status. The general recommendation is to eat more, but even a small amount, such as a fourth of a cup of blueberries, may promote good brain health.

10 Berries to Try:

▶ Blueberries: A superfood with many health benefits

▶ Blackberries: Related to raspberries; may be eaten fresh or in jams or preserves

▶ Strawberries: Popular red berry; eaten fresh or in jams or preserves

▶ Raspberries: Eaten fresh or in jams and preserves

▶ Black Currants: Round fruit often used in preserves or wines

▶ Lingonberries: Also known as cowberry; similar to cranberries

▶ Chokeberries: Often used in tarts and jams; grown wild throughout parts of the West

▶ Acai Berries: Dark purple fruit native to the Amazon jungle of South America

▶ Persimmons: These fruits with slightly mealy texture are botanically classified as berries

▶ Black Mulberries: Often used by cooks as a substitute for blackberries in wines or jams

91. THE DANGERS OF SUBSTANCE ABUSE

Substance abuse disorder is a major problem in the United States. Tobacco use, excessive alcohol intake, and illicit drugs have all contributed to destroyed lives, fractured relationships, financial challenges, decreased productivity, impaired cognitive function, poor health, and death. Because the problem of substance abuse is so significant and so complex, a multidisciplinary approach has to be used to effectively deal with it.

It is crucial that you address any substance abuse issues if you want have great health and live your best life.

10 Resources for Help with Substance Abuse:

- Alcoholics Anonymous: https://www.aa.org/

- SMART Recovery: https://www.smartrecovery.org/

- Women for Sobriety: https://womenforsobriety.org/

- WhoYouWant2Be.org

- Smokefree.gov

- 1-800-QUIT-NOW (smoking)

- American Lung Cancer Association: www.lung.org/stop-smoking

- Substance Abuse and Mental Health Services Administration: https://www.samhsa.gov/find-help/national-helpline

- Opioid Heroin Prevention Education Youth School Program: https://www.overdose-lifeline.org/opioid-heroin-prevention-education-program.html

- Narcotics Overdose Prevention and Education: http://www.nopetaskforce.org/about.php

THINGS TO HELP ME TRANSFORM

THINGS TO HELP ME TRANSFORM

_____

_____

_____

_____

_____

_____

_____

_____

_____

_____

_____

_____

_____

_____

_____

THINGS TO HELP ME TRANSFORM

THINGS TO HELP ME TRANSFORM

CHAPTER 8

Relationships

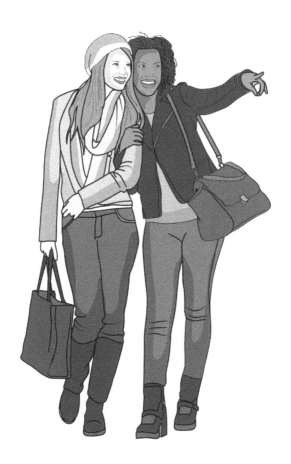

The most important things in life are the
connections you make with others.

~**Tom Ford**

92. STAY SOCIALLY CONNECTED

Staying socially connected is not only important to survival but appears to have a positive impact on one's health. There are also findings that suggest that decreased social connection may even play a role in compromising the immune function. Staying socially connected may be one of the best strategies to help decrease depression, isolation, and loneliness, which are often linked with various other diseases. For some people, loneliness can be as painful as physical pain. There is healing power in groups.

10 Strategies to Increase Social Connection:

▸ Go on a journey of self-discovery and reconnect with yourself.

▸ Make a list of family and friends and schedule a call or coffee each week.

▸ Join an in-person or online support group.

▸ Become involved in a community project.

▸ Volunteer.

▶ Create your own social network.

▶ Attend church or another supportive group.

▶ Get a pet.

▶ Work part-time.

▶ Enroll in a new fitness class or learn a new skill.

93.   IKIGAI

The term ikigai originates in the island of Okinawa Japan (said to be home to the largest population of centenarians in the world) and is often seen as the reason for living or your purpose. Ikigai is generally seen as a combination of your passion, mission, vocation, and profession. Discovering your own ikigai is said to bring fulfilment and happiness and make you live longer.

10 Strategies to Help You Achieve Your Ikigai:

▶ Surround yourself with good friends.

▶ Find work you enjoy.

▶ Look for balance in daily routine.

▶ Practice Morning Miracles.

▶ Stay active and don't retire.

▶ Live your life to leave a legacy.

▶ Eat healthily and keep physically active.

▶ Keep socially connected.

▶ Live in the present.

▶ Practice gratitude.

94. THE HAPPINESS HABIT

Happy, positive, and optimistic people not only enjoy better quality of life, they live longer as well. The current body of research suggests that happiness is linked to less cardiovascular disease, lower blood pressure, decreased likelihood of suffering from depression, and a greater life span.

Life won't always go your way, and sometimes you may experience very devastating situations. Even during these challenging times, you can choose how you respond, and you have the power to choose positivity.

10 Strategies to Increase your Happiness:

▶ Recognize that you are responsible for your own happiness.

▶ Look for the bright side of every disappointment.

▸ View challenges as the universe helping you to grow and learn.

▸ Know that at any moment you can change your attitude.

▸ Surround yourself with positive people.

▸ Limit pity parties to 10 minutes then move on.

▸ Decide how you want to feel and be proactive.

▸ Practice gratitude daily.

▸ Use kind words and be kind to yourself at all times.

▸ Find happiness in simple things such as the sunset, a cool breeze, or flowers.

THINGS TO HELP ME TRANSFORM

THINGS TO HELP ME TRANSFORM

THINGS TO HELP ME TRANSFORM

THINGS TO HELP ME TRANSFORM

_____

_____

_____

_____

_____

_____

_____

_____

_____

_____

_____

_____

_____

_____

_____

CHAPTER 9

Movement Is Medicine

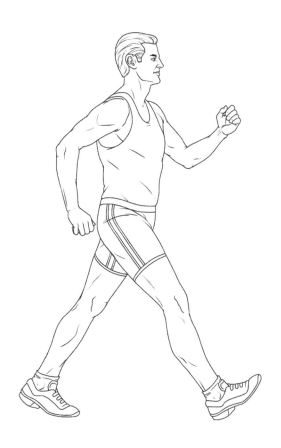

To enjoy the glow of good health, you must exercise.
~ **Gene Tunney**

95. THE BEST EXERCISE

The commonly asked question is what is the best exercise? The answer is the one you will actually do.

There are a variety of exercises available, including walking (my favorite), swimming, running, and Zumba. Exercise can also include the use of equipment, such as a treadmill, bikes, an elliptical, and weights. One way to help make the decision as to the best exercise for you includes the use of the S.S.A.F.F.E.E. acronym.

▸ Scientifically documented benefits: What does the research say about the activity?

▸ Safe: How safe is the exercise or equipment

▸ Appropriate to a person's unique needs and situation

▸ Functionally sound: How functional is the equipment?

▸ Feel or the experiential feel of the machine

▸ Effective: Will you achieve results?

▸ Enjoyment: Exercise can and should be fun

96.   SET A FITNESS PLAN AND GOAL

One of my favorite motivational speakers, Zig Ziglar, is credited with saying "You can't hit a target you cannot see, and you cannot see a target you do not have." My question to you is how can you achieve health goals you haven't defined?

Whenever you set out to achieve a goal or make health changes, it's imperative that you have a plan. A plan will serve as a blueprint for what you want to achieve and allows for periodic evaluation of that plan so you can see your progress.

A fitness goal allows you to state the results you hope to realize and is best achieved using the S.M.A.R.T. acronym. The acronym S.M.A.R.T. stands for

▶ Specific

▶ Measurable

▶ Achievable

▶ Realistic

▶ Time-sensitive

Instead of stating a general goals such as "I would like to lose weight," a more effective goal that passes the S.M.A.R.T. test would be "I will lose 10 pounds in the next 12 weeks (or by a specific date), and I will do this by taking a brisk 40-minute walk five times per week, decreasing my portion sizes, eating five servings of vegetables per day, and eliminating sodas and replacing them with sparkling water.

97. WAIST-TO-HIP RATIO

Waist-to-hip ratio (WHR) is a measure of the ratio of your waist circumference to your hip circumference and gives an indication of how much fat is stored in your waist, hips, and buttocks. The significance of this ratio is that is that people who carry more weight around their midsection (an apple shape) are at a higher risk than those who carry weight on their hips and thighs (a pear shape) for type 2 diabetes, heart disease, and death. This higher risk is still preset even when the body mass index (BMI) is normal.

A normal WHR in men is considered 0.9 or less and in women 0.85 or less. A WHR that is greater than 1.0 in either men or women is associated with a higher risk of cardiovascular disease. A high WHR may signify that it is time to get your health in order and to increase your exercise, improve your nutrition, get adequate sleep, reduce your stress, and improve your wellbeing.

Procedure for Measuring Your Waist-to-Hip Ratio

▶ Stand up straight and breathe out.

▶ Measure your waist circumference by using a tape measure to check the distance around the smallest part of your waist, just above your belly button.

▶ Measure your hip circumference by measuring the distance around the largest part of your hips or the widest part of your buttocks.

▶ Calculate your WHR by dividing your waist circumference by your hip circumference.

▶ Check to see if it is high, low, or normal.

98. CULTIVATE A MOVEMENT-BASED LIFESTYLE

When we examine the lifestyle practices of the people in the Blue Zones—the five places in the world where people live longer and healthier lives than average—we see that physical activity plays an integral role in their lives. Though most of these people don't have gym memberships, they all seem to have found ways to incorporate a movement-based lifestyle.

The current guidelines for exercise for Americans include at least 150 minutes of moderate activity or 75 minutes of vigorous activity per week spread out over the week and strength training at least two days per week. Since time constraint seems to be a limiting factor for many people achieving the recommendation, movement should always be included whenever possible. Add exercises such as walking, resistance training, flexibility training, high intensity training, aqua therapy, and tai chi into your routine.

10 Strategies for Cultivating a Movement-Based Lifestyle:

▶ Ask your doctor to write you an exercise prescription.

▶ Schedule the gym the same way you schedule an appointment.

▶ Get an accountability partner who is very physically active.

▶ Join the health challenges at your job.

▶ Park furthest away from the entrance and walk.

▶ Get off the train or bus one stop early and walk.

▶ Enroll in a physical activity class that meets at least twice weekly.

▶ Take the stairs instead of the elevator.

▶ Go to the mall early and walk from end to end.

▶ While at the airport waiting on a flight, set a timer and go for a walk.

99. THE EXERICSE PRESCRIPTION

Exercise is different from physical activities in that it is planned and structured. Because we know that exercise is medicine, your physician may write an exercise prescription in much the same way a prescription may be written for medications. The exercise prescription is a specific description of the exercise recommendations, and it uses the acronym FITT. The F stands for the frequency with which you are expected to perform the exercise. I stands for intensity and denotes low, medium, or high. T refers to the how much time should be spent doing the activity, and the final T specifies the type of activity.

Studies have shown that when exericse or food is prescribed, there is a greater likelihood the person who receives that prescription will comply. Since you know that health is your greatest wealth and exercise is medicine, why not ask your doctor about an exercise prescription?

Sample Exercise Prescription FITT Format:

Three times per week **(F)**, take a brisk **(I)** walk **(T)** for 45 minutes each session **(T)**.

100. THE POWER OF THE POSTURE

If you are like most people, you slouch. Maintaining good posture represents holding your body in a certain way while lying, sitting, standing, and walking so as to decease stress and strain on your ligaments, tendons, bones, muscles, and joints and to keep your body in good alignment.

5 Strategies for Good Posture:

▶ When standing, keep your chest out and your shoulders back.

▶ Stand up tall.

▶ Pull your chin back so your chest is centered over your shoulder.

▶ When sitting, distribute your body weight evenly on both hips.

▶ Sit up with your back straight and your shoulders back. Your buttocks should touch the back of your chair.

▶ Try to avoid sitting in the same position for more than 30 minutes.

▶ Avoid lifting heavy objects above waist level.

▶ To pick up an object that is lower than the level of your waist, keep your back straight and bend at your knees and hips.

▶ Hold packages close to your body with your arms bent. Keep your stomach muscles tight.

▶ Avoid sleeping on your stomach, especially on a saggy mattress, since this can cause back strain.

101. SITTING IS THE NEW SMOKING

As a child growing up in Jamaica, I was often admonished to "sit and keep still" or to "sit down." Now we know there is danger in prolonged sitting. There is a growing body of research showing an association between prolonged sitting and a myriad of illnesses, including heart disease, diabetes, and cancer. Sitting is now considered more dangerous than smoking and will kill more people than HIV. It is believed that prolonged sitting significantly can shorten your lifespan, shuts down the metabolism, contributes to obesity, prevents normal self-healing function of the body, and contributes to back pain. Another interesting piece of research shows that although exercise is great for you, it doesn't seem to change the negative effects of prolonged sitting.

The good thing is that the solution is easy. Get up and move and avoid prolonged sitting.

5 Strategies to Decrease Your Sitting Time:

▶ Use a standing desk.

▶ Use a desk treadmill.

▶ Set a timer and stand, stretch, and have some water every hour.

▶ While watching TV, instead of a chair, sit on a physio ball and engage your core.

▶ While on a plane, get up periodically. During seated times, do seated leg lifts.

THINGS TO HELP ME TRANSFORM

_____

_____

_____

_____

_____

_____

_____

_____

_____

_____

_____

_____

_____

_____

_____

_____

THINGS TO HELP ME TRANSFORM

THINGS TO HELP ME TRANSFORM

_____

_____

_____

_____

_____

_____

_____

_____

_____

_____

_____

_____

_____

_____

_____

_____

_____

THINGS TO HELP ME TRANSFORM

_____

_____

_____

_____

_____

_____

_____

_____

_____

_____

_____

_____

_____

_____

_____

_____

EPILOGUE

This ends the 101 lifestyle medicine and wellness practices that have the possibility of TRANSFORMing your health and life. I am grateful I was able to share these practices with you. I am also grateful to share my passion of helping people heal. I was unable to help my maternal grandfather and my father, who both died of preventable cardiopulmonary disease in their 50s; my maternal uncle, who suffered with diabetes and alcoholism; my paternal uncle, who had multiple strokes; and many other family members who have struggled with and died of lifestyle-related disorders. I am, however, in the fortunate position where I can help you and many others like you who have the potential to prevent these diseases, stop them in their tracks, or reverse them.

I would love to continue helping you and invite to contact me on my website at www.DrDianeThompson.com or on all social media at Dr. Diane Thompson. I also invite you to download the free e-book *8 Life-Changing Lifestyle Medicine and Wellness Tips* as shared by some of my former radio guests, who are also top experts in the country.

Remember, your health is your wealth, so do something healthy for yourself and your family.

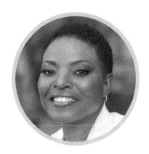

ABOUT THE AUTHOR

Dr. Diane Thompson is a triple board-certified physician, former nurse, certified health coach, certified yoga teacher, Complete Health Improvement Program (CHIP) facilitator, and award-winning speaker. She is the host of the popular and syndicated radio show *Health Talk with Dr. Diane MD* and the creator of the Healthy Inspiration Journal Series.

Dr. Thompson was born in Jamaica and moved to New York when she was sixteen. She was awarded the Sigma Theta Tau Honor Society's Award for Clinical Excellence, nominated for Physician of the Year, named New York SuperDoctors Rising Star 2018 and 2019, and has received numerous speaking awards.

Dr. Thompson enjoys reading, speaking, mentoring, writing, and listening to podcasts. She is married and resides in New York City.

Learn more at www.drdianethompson.com

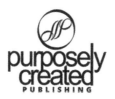